HYPNOSIS

Secrets of the Mind

HYPNOSIS
Secrets of the Mind

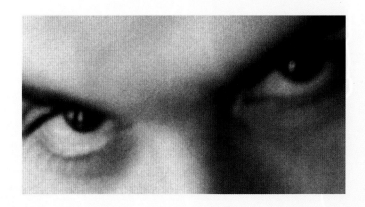

MICHAEL STREETER

BARRON'S

Contents

First edition for the United States, its territories and dependencies, and Canada, published in 2004 by Barron's Educational Series, Inc.

A QUARTO BOOK

All inquiries to be addressed to:
Barron's Educational Series, Inc.
250 Wireless Boulevard
Hauppauge, NY 11788
http://www.barronseduc.com

Library of Congress Catalog Card Number 2002117481

ISBN 0-7641-2593-1

QUAR.HYP

Conceived, designed, and produced by
Quarto Publishing plc
The Old Brewery
6 Blundell Street
London N7 9BH

Project Editors Fiona Robertson, Liz Pasfield
Art Editors Karla Jennings, Jill Mumford
Designer Maggie Aldred
Assistant Art Director Penny Cobb
Illustrator Mark Duffin
Photographer Paul Forrester
Text Editor Andrew Armitage
Proofreader Anne Plume
Art director Moira Clinch
Publisher Piers Spence

Manufactured by PICA Digital, Singapore
Printed by Midas International printing, China
9 8 7 6 5 4 3 2 1

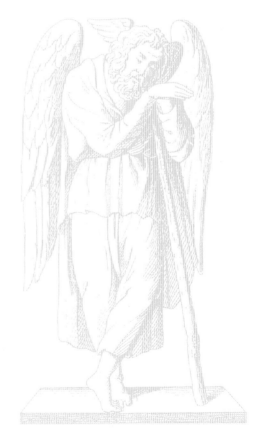

Introduction

Mention the word "hypnosis" to someone and the chances are you will get one of three very different reactions: intense curiosity, nervousness, or disdainful skepticism. Hypnosis has attracted all three responses since it first began to excite scientific interest in the eighteenth century.

For those who are convinced that humans have within them vast reservoirs of untapped potential, hypnosis is a source of great fascination. What could be more natural than harnessing the full power of the human mind?

Yet for others the very idea of delving deep into the hidden corners of our minds seems to be asking for trouble. For them, hypnosis is mysterious, secretive, and even dangerous. Is it not linked with the occult and un-Christian?

The third group—the skeptics—scoff at a subject rejected by many rational scientists for the last two centuries. Why should we take seriously a phenomenon that is historically the stuff of showmen, quacks, and occultists?

The skeptics are right about one thing at least: hypnosis is about the imagination. The story of hypnosis is also about humanity's unending quest to explore the inner workings of the most powerful thing we possess—our minds.

Hypnosis: Secrets of the Mind tackles head-on the fears and the doubts that have plagued hypnosis for more than 200 years. It charts the extraordinary history of hypnotism, describes what it is and how it works, and details the variety of practical and beneficial treatments that modern hypnotists now provide. By the end, this book will have provided you with the chance to make use of this incredibly powerful technique yourself— thanks to self-hypnosis.

Along the way, the book also explores some of the darker side of hypnosis and mind control—how, for example, the CIA tried to use hypnotism to create assassins, amid fears that communist regimes were using hypnosis on American prisoners of war. And how some hypnotic stage acts of the past have gone horribly wrong.

For there is no doubting that the public image of hypnosis has suffered from a checkered past. One of the eighteenth-century founding fathers of hypnosis, Franz Anton Mesmer, was widely regarded by his peers as a fraud, and the

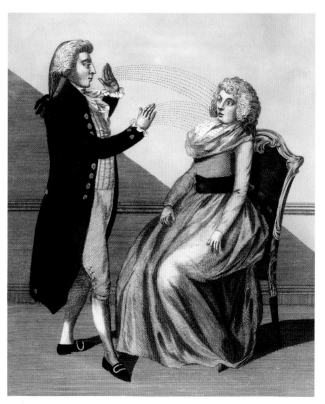

ᒰIn eighteenth-century forms of hypnosis, experts tried to hypnotize their clients by what were called "mesmeric passes." In the early years nearly all patients were women.

more lurid fears surrounding hypnosis can be traced back to his time. His practice of laying his hands on his (mostly female) patients to impart his "animal magnetism" was bound to invite accusations of impropriety. The scurrilous image of hypnotism reached its peak in 1894, when George du Maurier published a novel on the subject. Few people now know the name of the book—*Trilby*—but most will recognize the name of the sinister character who is the novel's antihero—Svengali. For more than 100 years, the name Svengali has been synonymous with evil staring eyes, the control of helpless women, and hypnosis.

Helpful Hypnosis

Yet beyond these clichés lies a wonderful world of beneficial hypnosis. We will see how the therapy is used today to quit smoking, lose weight, pass tests, relieve pain, and remove phobias. In the last half-century, the scientific and medical establishments have realized that hypnosis is not to be dismissed as worthy only of the stage or of parlor games. Instead, it is now seen as a powerful therapeutic tool that is being adopted in more and more hospitals.

⤸The writer George du Maurier should take much of the blame for the bad public image of hypnosis with his creation of the fictional character Svengali. Modern hypnotists are still working to overcome this negative stereotype of how hypnosis works.

Scientists may still differ about the exact nature of hypnosis, but what hypnosis actually involves is no great mystery—and nothing to cause alarm. The conscious, critical mind is bypassed or distracted. This allows the ever-present unconscious or subconscious mind to dominate in the state we call hypnotic trance. The unconscious mind is the repository of our beliefs, imagination, fears, and associations. Influence this, and we can change our unconscious reaction to the world around us. This is what happens in hypnosis: changes are suggested to the unconscious mind, which then acts upon these suggestions. The amazing part is that it really seems to work.

The technique has allowed people with phobias to overcome them, has enabled women to give birth with little or no pain, and has helped students to take exams without anxiety. Top sportsmen and women, as well as leaders and celebrities, have turned to hypnosis to achieve their goals and improve their lives, along with many thousands of ordinary people of all backgrounds and beliefs. Of course, hypnosis is not a miracle cure. We will never be able to run 100 meters in 10 seconds or win the Nobel Prize for literature just because we have undergone hypnosis. But what it can do is help to unlock our individual potential.

The scientific and medical view has tilted back in favor of hypnosis; the public perception is still lagging a little behind. Soon, however, we will all begin to realize our true power, and the way that hypnosis can harness the ability that resides in us all.

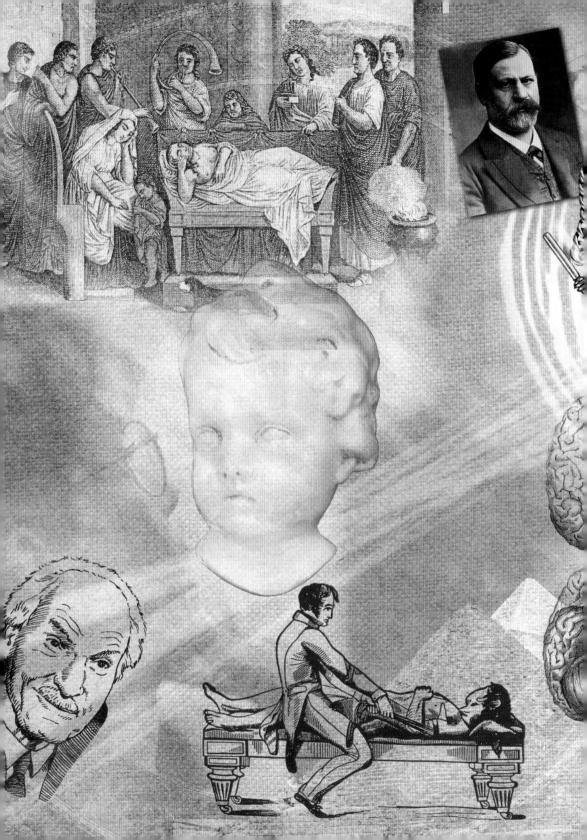

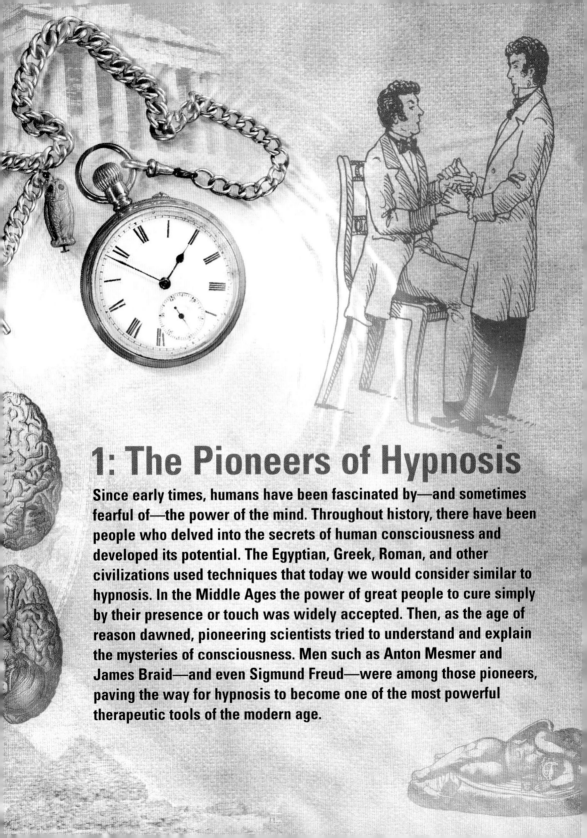

1: The Pioneers of Hypnosis

Since early times, humans have been fascinated by—and sometimes fearful of—the power of the mind. Throughout history, there have been people who delved into the secrets of human consciousness and developed its potential. The Egyptian, Greek, Roman, and other civilizations used techniques that today we would consider similar to hypnosis. In the Middle Ages the power of great people to cure simply by their presence or touch was widely accepted. Then, as the age of reason dawned, pioneering scientists tried to understand and explain the mysteries of consciousness. Men such as Anton Mesmer and James Braid—and even Sigmund Freud—were among those pioneers, paving the way for hypnosis to become one of the most powerful therapeutic tools of the modern age.

The roots of hypnotism

The fascinating story of hypnosis can be traced back to the ancient world. The Egyptians seem to have used a form of healing in which priests spoke and laid hands on patients while they were "asleep"—or at least had their eyes closed. This intriguing technique was practiced at least 3000 years ago. The ancient Chinese and Indian civilizations are also thought to have performed a kind of healing in which words, and words alone, were used to help cure patients.

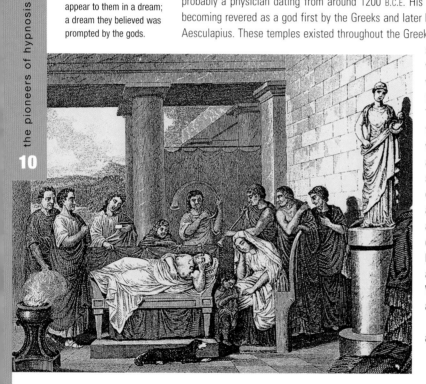

◁In the ancient world physicians used what are known as temples of sleep, in which the patient would be encouraged to spend a night. As they slept the cure for their illness would appear to them in a dream; a dream they believed was prompted by the gods.

The Greeks, meanwhile, had what are sometimes called temples of sleep, in which patients desperate for a cure would lie down and sleep. The idea was that, as the patient slept, the cure for his or her ailment would appear in a dream. The most popular of these temples was the one dedicated to the Greek god of healing, Asclepius. Asclepius was probably a physician dating from around 1200 B.C.E. His prowess as a healer led to his becoming revered as a god first by the Greeks and later by the Romans, who called him Aesculapius. These temples existed throughout the Greek world and were regarded as a standard and perfectly normal way of seeking treatment. It was believed that the gods implanted the idea for the cure. This cure would either work then and there, or the patient would have to go away and administer it himself. In one story, a man who was blind in one eye sought help—apparently to much skepticism at the time. As the patient slept, one of the gods appeared to him, boiled some herbs, and applied them to the bad eye. When he awoke the man was able to see with it.

We must, however, be careful about regarding these sleep

c. 3000 B.C.E.

c. 2600 B.C.E.: The father of Chinese medicine, Wong Tai, writes about healing techniques that involved using words to help cure people.

c. 2500 B.C.E.   c. 2000 B.C.E.   c. 1500 B.C.E.

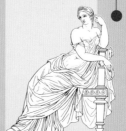

c. 1200 B.C.E.: The Greek physician Asclepius carries out healing; later he is worshiped as the god of healing. Greeks, then Romans, develop temples of sleep, where patients are told of their cure while dreaming.

temples and other ancient practices as hypnosis as we understand it. The key elements—the deliberate inducing of a trance and then using suggestions to the unconscious mind—were certainly not practiced in the way modern hypnotists perform them. However, these examples show that the ancients may well have understood the power of the mind and imagination to effect cures, the basic ingredients of hypnosis.

The Royal Touch

The power of the mind and imagination was also important in another healing process of the past. This was the famed ability of great people, for example, kings, to be able to cure people simply by the power of touch. One such man was the Greek leader King Pyrrhus of Epirus (318–272 B.C.E.). He is best known for the two victories he won over the Romans at such huge cost to his own side that they were not worth winning; hence the expression a "Pyrrhic victory." Pyrrhus, though, had another claim to fame: the touch of his big toe was supposed to cure illness. At least two Roman emperors, Vespasian (9–79 C.E.) and Hadrian (76–138 C.E.), were renowned for similar powers, although not with their feet. Nearer our own times, the English king Edward the Confessor (1003–1066) and his near contemporary Philip I of France were credited with the ability to heal by touch. These examples hint at what we might now call the power of suggestion. That is, patients become convinced in their minds that they are going to be cured, and this in turn helps the body to heal itself. The belief that royalty, clergy, and other dignitaries could cure simply by touching someone lasted through the Middle Ages and into more modern times. The British monarch King Charles II (1630–1685) used the "Royal Touch" thousands of times during his reign.

King Charles II ↵

Valentine Greatrakes

Valentine Greatrakes (1628–1682) was known as "The Stroker" because of his apparent ability to heal people with the touch of his hands. During the seventeenth century, the Irish-born soldier and government official attracted considerable fame because of his powers, and was apparently able to cure a number of ailments including scrofula—a disfiguring skin disease—and warts. Interestingly, some of his patients appeared to go into a deep trancelike state during his treatment, at which time they could feel no pain. This has parallels with modern hypnosis, in which some patients experience analgesia—insensibility to pain—during a trance. Greatrakes's reputation attracted the attention of some men of science at the time, and also of the British king, Charles II. His main technique appeared to be touching the patient, through his or her clothing, though he sometimes used potions as well. It is possible that Greatrakes in effect "hypnotized" his patients without realizing it and their minds acted upon the implicit suggestion that they were being cured.

---

c. 1000 B.C.E.

● c. 1000 B.C.E.: Egyptians have temples where priests carry out healing by word and touch.

c. 500 B.C.E.

● c. 300 B.C.E.: King Pyrrhus of Epirus is able to cure by the touch of his big toe.

c. 100 B.C.E.

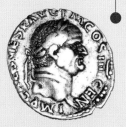

● c. 70 C.E.: The Roman emperor Vespasian is said to be able to cure by the power of touch.

Imagination and Magnets

The Royal Touch phenomenon was taken seriously. During the Middle Ages, academics and great thinkers contemplated how the power of the mind, and particularly imagination and will, could have an impact on the healing process. One fourteenth-century writer, Peter of Abano, considered that patients could be successfully treated simply by the use of will alone. Later, Georg Pictorius von Villingen (1500–1569) claimed that the use of spells or incantations to cure people could be more effective if both healer and patient used imagination. This theory sounds similar to what we now call the placebo effect, which brings about a cure even though no medication as such has been taken, but only, in some cases, a sugar pill. The effect is brought about by the mind's power over the body, because the patient believes a "real" pill has been swallowed.

Another from that era to champion the power of the imagination was the Swiss-born physician, scientist, and alchemist Paracelsus (Theophrastus Bombastus von Hohenheim, 1493–1541). Paracelsus was one of the earliest pioneers of medicine to advocate the use of chemical and mineral treatments for illnesses. He was also very aware of the power of the mind, describing imagination as an "instrument" of healing. Paracelsus maintained that, "The moral atmosphere surrounding the patient can have a strong influence on the course of the disease. It is not the curse or the blessing that works, but the idea. The imagination produces the effect." Imagination was not everything.

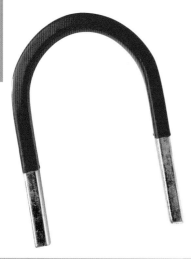

⟨The mysterious properties of magnets and magnetism were applied to the human body by early thinkers such as the sixteenth-century scientist Paracelsus. He firmly believed that magnets could attract diseases out of people in the same way they attracted metal.

Father Hell

Paracelsus's theory that magnets could attract diseases in the way they attract iron was developed by a number of scientists in later centuries. The idea was that the body contained a magnetic fluid, and that illness could be caused by a defect in that fluid. Magnets could cure it.

One man who took up this idea in the eighteenth century was an astronomer and priest who rejoiced in the name of Father Maximilian Hell (1720–1792). Hell was a distinguished scientist and became director of the Imperial Observatory in Vienna, then capital of the Austro-Hungarian Empire. He was also fascinated by Paracelsus's idea of using magnetism to cure people. The discovery in the middle of the eighteenth century that magnets could be made artificially contributed to a surge of interest in this treatment. Hell discovered that, by arranging magnets in certain ways around a patient, he could cure or relieve a number of ailments, including rheumatism, from which he himself suffered. Though Hell seems to have

1000

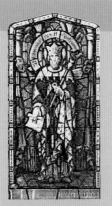

c. 1060: The English king Edward the Confessor is said to have had the power to cure by touching.

1100

c. 1100: King Philip I of France is reputed to have healing powers in his hands.

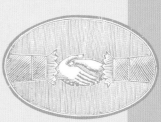

1200

1300

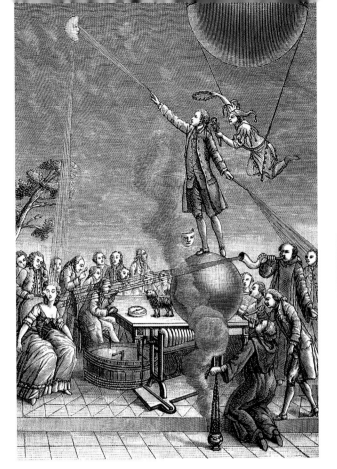

⌄The eighteenth century was full of self-appointed experts and showmen who claimed they could cure patients with a range of exotic techniques, including the use of magnets and magnetism. One of these was a priest who had the unforgettable name of Maximilian Hell.

been quite successful with his treatments, he would have had no place in the history of hypnosis had his services not been called upon by another medical man in Vienna in 1774. That man was Franz Anton Mesmer. The story of modern hypnosis was about to begin.

Father Gassner

This Catholic priest from Switzerland was a colorful character who briefly became famous during the 1770s as a great healer. Father Gassner (1727–1779) believed that he could cure people by releasing the evil spirits that were in their bodies. A natural showman, he wore a long cloak, carried a large crucifix, and spoke Latin incantations during his immensely popular "shows." He told his patients that they would fall to the ground and then "die" while he carried out his exorcism. Then, once the spirits were gone, the patients would come back to life and find themselves completely cured. Oddly enough, people did seem to be cured by this. The priest's technique foreshadows the hypnotic methods of putting people into a trance, then using the power of suggestion to assert that their ailments or problems have disappeared. Father Gassner, however, believed his work was all about using God to drive out evil spirits. One of the people asked to report on Father Gassner's methods was Franz Anton Mesmer, who decided that the priest was unwittingly using animal magnetism.

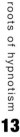

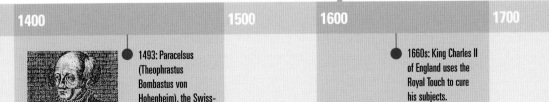

1400

1500

1600

1700

1493: Paracelsus (Theophrastus Bombastus von Hohenheim), the Swiss-born academic who believed that a form of magnetism controls our health, is born.

1660s: King Charles II of England uses the Royal Touch to cure his subjects.

Franz Anton Mesmer

Most of us have heard the terms "mesmerizing" and "mesmeric." Both words come from Franz Anton Mesmer, who was born in 1734 near Lake Constance, close to the modern border between Germany and Switzerland. Mesmer was a slightly odd, even eccentric man who was regarded by many in his day as a fraud. By today's standards, he certainly had some strange theories. But Mesmer is nevertheless viewed as one of the most important personalities in the history of hypnotism. Ironically, Mesmer never appeared to understand the true power of the mind, and would have rejected current thinking on the subject. Yet his fame, charisma, and apparent effectiveness at curing patients ultimately encouraged later pioneers on their path to understanding the true nature of hypnosis.

The son of a gamekeeper, the young Mesmer studied theology, and then law, before gravitating toward the subject that was to make his name and fortune—medicine. He graduated from the prestigious Medical School in Vienna in 1765. The young doctor had a strong interest in the planets and in phenomena such as the tides. This led him to study the effects of external influences on the human body. His thesis at the university

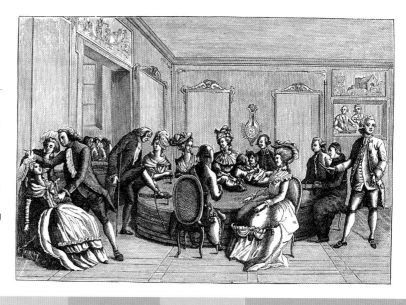

↳Mesmer's healing sessions were often public affairs and the controversial character was as much a showman as a physician. His patients were arranged around a bath filled with iron filings and water, which Mesmer claimed helped to create the mesmeric healing effect. Once patients had undergone a "crisis" they were cured.

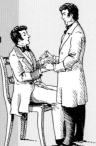

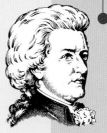

1730   1740   1750   1760   1770

1734: Franz Anton Mesmer is born on May 23 at Iznang, in what is now Germany.

1770s: Mesmer practices as a successful doctor in Vienna, and is a friend of Leopold Mozart and his brilliant musician son Wolfgang.

suggested, as other scientists had done before, that there existed some kind of universal gravitational fluid. This fluid was the medium through which, for example, large objects such as planets were able to exert influence on other objects, including the human body. Though this may seem peculiar to us now, it was not an original or particularly weird view at that time. It was, though, the start of his exploration of what became known as "animal magnetism."

A Meeting with Hell

At first Mesmer practiced as an ordinary doctor in Vienna, where he lived a comfortable life thanks to his marriage to a wealthy widow, Maria Anna von Posch. It was at that time that he befriended the young and precocious composer Wolfgang Amadeus Mozart, and the doctor and his wife moved in the highest circles. Then in 1774 events occurred that were to change Mesmer's life forever. One of his patients, Francisca Oesterlin, had failed to respond to conventional treatment for her nervous complaints, and out of curiosity he decided to try the unorthodox methods used by one of his contemporaries—Father Maximilian Hell. Mesmer asked Oesterlin to drink a liquid containing some iron and then attached magnets to her body. After a seizure, and several sessions of treatment, the patient was cured.

For Mesmer, this was a turning point. He was convinced he had discovered the power of magnetism. Soon, he was adapting his old theories about a universal fluid to his newfound passion. Mesmer now claimed there existed a universal magnetic fluid that connected everything—including people—and developed his theory called animal magnetism. (In this context "animal" means "vital" or "live" rather than relating to a mammal or other creature.) He became convinced that disease was caused by blockages in the flow of the magnetism through a person's body. Mesmer would now use magnets to influence the magnetic fluids in a patient's body, remove the blockages, and help cure disease.

Mesmer's Views

Mesmer believed that there was a physical explanation for the cures he could effect using magnets and iron rods. He thought that there was a universal magnetic fluid, and that something similar existed inside our bodies. By manipulating

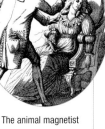
The animal magnetist

this magnetic fluid, Mesmer believed he could cure various disorders, including nervous conditions. He also maintained that it was his own powerful animal magnetism that helped influence this process, and that he was passing this on to the patient. His aim was to establish a "magnetic polarity" between healer and patient. The fact that Mesmer touched his patients as part of this process, and that nearly all were women, caused some critics to suspect his motives. His patients also often went through convulsions and crises during the sessions.

It is one of the great ironies that Mesmer, who is rightly held up as an early pioneer of hypnosis, firmly believed that the cause of his cures was physical and not psychological; that is, he believed it was magnetism that helped the patient. In his treatments he gave little weight to the role of the patient's mind or imagination, one of the cornerstones of modern hypnosis.

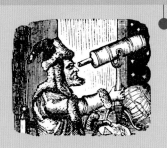

1774: A Jesuit priest, Maximilian Hell, who was the royal astronomer in Vienna, Austria, uses hypnotic techniques and metal plates. Mesmer borrows the same technique to cure a patient. He discovers animal magnetism.

c. 1775–1776: A priest, Father Gassner, performs a form of stage hypnosis. His shows are witnessed by Mesmer, who claims Gassner is using animal magnetism.

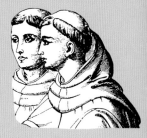

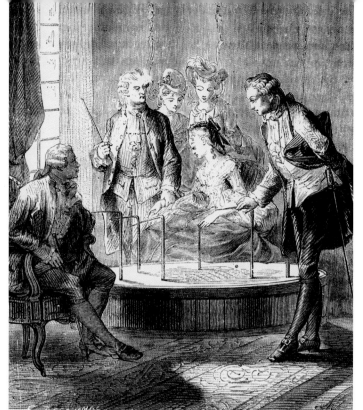

↪Mesmer's most controversial patient was a young blind musician called Maria Theresa Paradis who was a favorite of the Austrian empress. Her blindness at first began to disappear following his treatment but then returned; the resulting public furor forced Mesmer to quit Vienna for Paris.

The Blind Musician

Mesmer soon became a celebrity thanks to his new treatment. The rich and famous, especially women, flocked to see him, and his treatments took society by storm as his sessions became shows. That was not all, for he also offered his services free to the poor, and helped women endure the pain of childbirth. Mesmer's fame was at its height. The scientific community, however, was less convinced and viewed the doctor's methods with suspicion. The case that caused Mesmer's woes involved a singer and pianist in Vienna named Maria Theresa Paradis, who was just 18 at the time and a favorite of the empress. Maria had also been blind since she was a young girl. Mesmer took the young woman on as his patient in 1777 after the efforts of eminent doctors at the time to restore her sight had ended in failure. Using his bizarre equipment of metal and glass rods and baths filled with water and iron filings, which apparently focused the magnetic flows, Mesmer started treating the young woman. The treatment seems to have had an effect and according to Mesmer her eyesight did begin to return. Unfortunately for Mesmer, however, this very success was to prove his undoing. Jealous and well-connected doctors who had failed to help the teenager encouraged her parents to take the girl away from Mesmer's care. Maria's blindness, which may have been caused by a nonphysical, hysterical condition, promptly returned and Mesmer's reputation was tarnished. The frustrated and angry doctor was forced to leave Vienna and head for Paris.

1770

1780

1778: Rejected by the Austrian scientific community after the controversy of the case of Maria von Paradis, Franz Mesmer moves from Vienna to Paris.

1784: Benjamin Franklin heads a committee of inquiry set up by King Louis XVI in Paris to examine Mesmer's claims. He dismisses the phenomenon of mesmerism and animal magnetism as all in the mind.

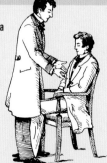

1784: Armand, Marquis de Puységur, a former student of Mesmer, discovers a form of deep trance he calls somnambulism.

For a while, Mesmer also found the French capital a fruitful place for his unusual ideas. The queen herself—Marie Antoinette—is said to have taken an interest in his work, yet his outlandish theories soon landed him in trouble again. Leading scientists insisted Mesmer was a fraud and that the flourishing practice of mesmerism was mere trickery. To settle the issue, King Louis XVI set up a committee in 1784 to investigate the claims of animal magnetism. Its disparaging verdict that animal magnetism did not exist was a heavy blow for Mesmer.

Rejected once more by the scientific community, the unfortunate doctor left Paris and started traveling, still convinced of his theories and still treating patients, yet unable to persuade the scientific community of his worth. He died, in relative though comfortable obscurity, near his home village in 1815.

Mesmer's Legacy

Why is Mesmer, a discredited, eccentric doctor, now so prominent in the story of hypnotism? His legacy is that, without him even realizing it, he had hit upon the importance and power of suggestion on patients who are in a trance. The rods, magnets, and iron filings that Mesmer used in his treatments were in themselves ineffective. But they may have helped focus patients' minds, and may have made them open to the implicit suggestion that they were going to be cured by the treatment. This, it seems, is why Mesmer's treatment worked in practice, even if his theory of why it worked was wrong. Soon, other physicians interested in Mesmer's methods began to realize that it was not the magnets or animal magnetism that were the key to success, but the power of the mind. So, while Mesmer may himself have been eccentric and misguided, it was his work in this area that helped open the door to others. His achievements encouraged them to explore the true power of the mind—and ultimately of hypnosis.

Benjamin Franklin and the Committee on Mesmerism

In 1784 the French government under King Louis XVI set up a committee to investigate Mesmer's theories of animal magnetism. The membership of the committee reads like a *Who's Who* of the great and good of the day. They included Dr. Joseph Ignace Guillotin, the man who gave his name to the instrument of execution called the guillotine, and Antoine Laurent Lavoisier, the famous chemist. Meanwhile the committee was headed by the American ambassador to Paris at the time, none other than Benjamin Franklin, the American statesman and famous scientist.

Benjamin Franklin

Unfortunately for Mesmer, this illustrious committee concentrated more on the scientist's theories than on his clinical success. They also tried to test how much magnetism one could add to a tree—Mesmer claimed he could magnetize inanimate objects—with predictable results. The committee concluded that "magnetic fluid" did not exist and that Mesmer's work was a sham.

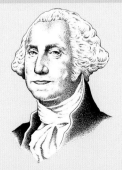

c. 1785: The Marquis de Lafayette tries but fails to impress George Washington with the benefits of mesmerism.

1808: British surgeon and proponent of the use of hypnosis in surgery, James Esdaile, is born.

The Marquis and magnetic sleep

The interest in animal magnetism did not disappear after the death of Mesmer. In the provinces, away from the scientific establishments of the capital cities, the fascination with the subject continued as enthusiasts, free from skeptical gaze, made new discoveries. One of the most important of these pioneers was an aristocratic French landowner, the Marquis de Puységur (1751–1825). The marquis had briefly been a student of Mesmer's techniques and later tried them out on workers on his estate situated northeast of Paris. To the marquis' astonishment, he found he was able to put a young shepherd named Victor Race into a sleeplike state during which the pair could still converse (see page 19). The marquis had apparently discovered the hypnotic trance. The aristocrat had certainly not been aiming to achieve this, because, as a loyal student of Mesmer, he assumed that the subject would suffer a crisis and convulsions. The marquis called this state somnambulism—a term familiar in modern hypnosis—or "magnetic sleep," in deference to Mesmer's ideas. Soon, however, Mesmer's former pupil began to doubt the existence of magnetic fluid as the basis of this phenomenon. Instead, de

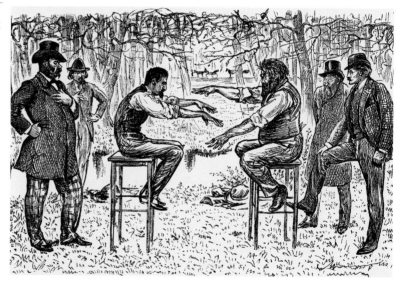

⌒The power of animal magnetism and mesmerism caught the public imagination, as shown by this Mesmeric "duel" in the Bois de Boulogne in the nineteenth century.

1810

1814: A Portuguese priest, Abbé Faria, develops the theory of suggestion and autosuggestion, and realizes the key to hypnotism: that everything takes place in the subject's mind, not in the mind of the mesmerist.

1815: Mesmer dies close to the village where he was born, largely forgotten by the scientific community.

1820

1821: First reports are heard of painless dentistry and surgery in France using magnetism.

1826: A French scientific commission gives qualified backing to mesmerism.

1830

Puységur put his emphasis on two important qualities—will and belief. A healer with both these qualities could succeed. This idea led him away from the baths, iron rods, and other paraphernalia that Mesmer and others had used, as well as from the crises and convulsions his mentor induced. Another of the marquis' important contributions was that he entered into conversations with his patients while they were in their sleeplike states, and suggested solutions to their problems. This marks the origins of hypnotherapy.

Following de Puységur's findings, other practitioners of magnetism found they could induce this sleeplike state, as well as discovering other conditions known to modern hypnotists, such as catalepsy (temporary inability to move a part of the body during a trance) and amnesia. Though not well known today, de Puységur is one of the unsung heroes in the development of hypnosis.

Abbè Jose di Faria

Gradually, the ideas of magnetism were spreading, though the belief that it was a physical process based on the passing of magnetic fluid from healer to patient was diminishing. Instead, more emphasis was being placed on the use of will and of the mind. The Portuguese priest, Abbè Jose di Faria (1753–1816), took this further. Di Faria was a showman, but he did come up with two important points in the development of hypnosis. The priest's technique was to get his subjects to stare at a fixed object, usually his hand. This method of hypnotic induction became familiar in later years. Second, di Faria emphasized the importance of the sleeplike state (trance) as the time when the mind is open to suggestions. This too is a key feature of modern hypnosis.

However, the scientific establishment in France—one of the centers of science in the world at the time—remained resolutely unimpressed by the claims of magnetism. For a while, the story of hypnotism switched elsewhere.

Victor Race

In 1783 the Marquis de Puységur tried his newly learned methods of animal magnetism on a 23-year-old shepherd named Victor Race, who worked on his estate. Initially the marquis used "magnetic passes"—touching the young man with his hands to help channel the magnetic fluid he believed was central to the technique. To his surprise, Victor fell into a sleeplike state, which the marquis later called magnetic sleep or somnambulism. The aristocrat had discovered trance. He found that Victor was able to converse during the trance and appeared more confident than in his waking state. De Puységur was able to put his subject into this state, and bring him out of it, at will, and developed a great rapport with both Victor and other subjects. The marquis also "magnetized" an elm tree on his estate and tied ropes to it, which other workers held. He found that some of these, too, fell into the sleeplike state. This story became so famous that other landowners had to "magnetize" trees on their estates to keep their workers happy. The marquis had discovered that hypnosis did not depend on magnets or convulsions, as his one-time teacher Mesmer believed. Instead, it relied on a close rapport between healer and patient, and, most importantly, the inducing of this sleeplike trance state.

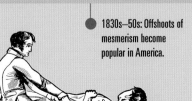

1830s: John Elliotson, president of the Royal Medical and Surgical Society of London, shows an interest in animal magnetism and uses trances to perform 1,834 surgical operations.

1830s–50s: Offshoots of mesmerism become popular in America.

1836: A teenage boy in Boston has a tooth extracted while under hypnosis.

1837: A second French commission rejects the therapeutic claims of mesmerism.

Surgery and quackery

One of the most fascinating and also controversial uses of early hypnosis was as a kind of anesthetic to stop a patient's pain during an operation. British doctor James Esdaile, who tried the technique in India, saw the post-operative death rate at his hospital fall from 50 to 5 percent after using hypnosis on patients undergoing surgery.

One of the more remarkable characters in the history of hypnosis is a Scottish surgeon by the name of James Esdaile (1808–1859). Esdaile worked in the 1840s at a hospital in Calcutta, India, then part of the British Empire. One of the problems with surgery at that time was that there was no effective anesthesia. The pain and discomfort of operations therefore ensured a high mortality rate. Esdaile's solution was to use mesmerism, as it was still called widely then, to induce anesthesia in his patients. (This should not come as a surprise: hypnosis is sometimes used today in surgery, notably in dental work, in place of chemical anesthetics. See page 76.) Esdaile had heard about this unorthodox technique from Europe and decided he had little to lose by using it. The results were impressive. More than 3000 operations using hypnosis were carried out at his hospital (by Esdaile and other doctors), and the post-operative death rate fell from around 50 percent to just 5 percent. One of the most remarkable operations was the removal of a man's tumor, which weighed an amazing 103 pounds (46.7 kg). The patient made a full recovery and claimed to have felt no pain during the growth's removal. However, Esdaile's

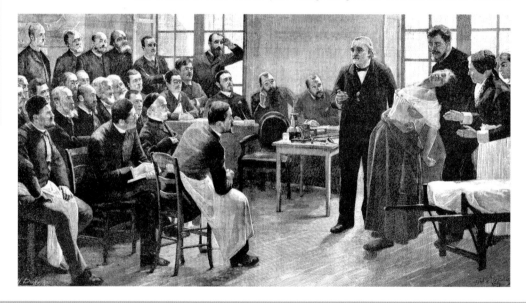

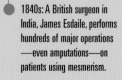

1840s: A British surgeon in India, James Esdaile, performs hundreds of major operations —even amputations—on patients using mesmerism.

1840: The Magnetic Society is formed in New Orleans to study hypnosis and its effects.

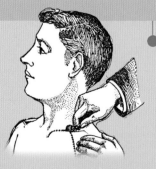

1841: A Scottish eye doctor and physician, James Braid, sees a demonstration of mesmerism and later uses it to perform pain-free surgery.

considerable success did not herald a breakthrough in the surgical use of hypnosis. His methods were regarded with suspicion by many of his fellow Europeans in India. Moreover, at around this time, in the 1840s, the arrival of ether and then chloroform became the established way to produce anesthesia.

Back in Britain, the medical use of mesmerism was viewed with equal suspicion. One of the main targets of skepticism was a physician named John Elliotson (1791–1868). Elliotson is an important figure in the history of hypnosis because, when he became interested in the subject, he was already a highly respected figure in the medical world. The fact that so eminent a person championed the cause of magnetism ensured that the subject was hotly debated in medical circles in Britain, even if ultimately he was fighting a lost cause. The doctor was introduced to the mysteries of magnetism by a Frenchman, Baron Dupotet, in the 1830s. As a result of what he saw, Elliotson began to use the technique to treat patients with nervous disorders, and as an anesthetic during surgery, at University College Hospital, London, where he was the senior physician. His method was to pass a piece of magnetized metal, such as nickel, over the patient's body in what were called magnetic or mesmeric passes. Elliotson, who had already written a standard medical textbook on more orthodox matters, reported great results from his use of mesmerism, which he believed to be a purely physical process and not psychological. In one case he claimed a woman made a full recovery from breast cancer after a number of sessions. Yet once again in the story of hypnosis, the medical establishment turned its back on the idea. It was rejected not because it did not work but because no one could properly explain it.

Mesmeric Mania

Though the medical establishment was mostly disdainful of mesmerism, much of society was captivated by some of the mesmeric performances that were given in the 1840s and 1850s. Indeed, 1851 was called a time of "mesmeric mania" in Britain. From the 1830s until the early 1850s, there was indeed an explosion of interest in the subject, thanks to huge numbers of books, pamphlets, newspaper and magazine articles, and traveling performers. Mesmerists traveled around the country giving shows to packed audiences, the performances mixing lectures on the subject with more show business elements such as young girls apparently lifting 200-pound (90.7kg) men or hypnotized boys playing cards while blindfolded. Well-known figures such as Charles Dickens were fascinated by the subject, and the author Charlotte Brontë was once mesmerized. So for 20 years mesmerism was a hot subject. There was also an air of sexual danger about mesmerism, with the continuing suspicion that men could use the exotic technique to gain power over a virtuous but defenseless woman. Eventually, though, the new craze gave way to other passions, including the Victorian fascination with the occult.

⤿The popularity of hypnosis during the nineteenth century touched all sections of society. Famous writers such as Charles Dickens took an interest in the phenomenon.

1850   1860   1870   1880

1843: Braid publishes a book in which he renames mesmerism "hypnosis" from the Greek name for the god of sleep, Hypnos.

1851: This is the year of "mesmeric mania" in Britain.

1885: Sigmund Freud works under French neurologist Jean-Martin Charcot, who uses hypnosis in his Paris clinic. Freud becomes a public champion of hypnosis.

The father of hypnosis

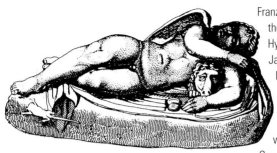

Franz Anton Mesmer may be the best-known name in the history of hypnosis, but the accolade of Father of Hypnosis should really go to the Scottish physician James Braid. Braid (1795–1860) was everything that Mesmer was not. He was a hard-headed practical man, methodical in his approach to science and not given to showmanship or hyperbole. One enduring achievement was Braid's invention of the word "hypnosis," adapting it from the name of the Greek god of sleep, Hypnos. He later realized, though, that the use of a word meaning "sleep" was not the best choice. Just as important, Braid was very clear about what hypnosis was—and what it was not. He rejected the idea of magnetic fluid and magnetism, which had come from Mesmer, and instead saw hypnosis as essentially psychological in nature.

Braid was working in Manchester, England, in 1841 when his interest in the subject began. He attended a show given by the flamboyant French mesmerist Charles de Lafontaine and was initially skeptical. However, at a later private meeting with Lafontaine and colleagues, at which the Frenchman put his subjects into a deep trance, Braid became convinced that there was a real scientific phenomenon to investigate. So anxious was Braid to understand what he had seen that after just two years of experiments with mesmerism he published his own book on the subject, *Neurypnology*. It was in this 1843 book that he used the term "hypnotism" for the first time.

Braid was the first real modern hypnotist. He did not associate the phenomenon with the occult; he did not believe it was caused by magnetic fluid or animal magnetism.

↶Though the word "hypnosis" is associated with the Greek word for sleep, the description is misleading. During hypnotic trances patients are not asleep; instead their unconscious minds are in a state of heightened awareness— a bit like when we daydream.

⌐In 1931 the actor John Barrymore gave a mesmerizing performance as George du Maurier's hypnotic antihero in the movie *Svengali*.

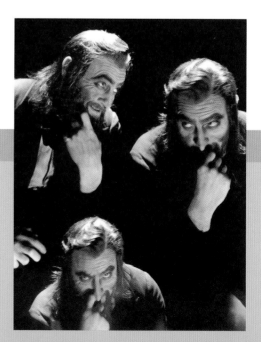

1890

● 1892: The British Medical Association reports favorably on the use of hypnosis in medicine.

● 1894: George du Maurier publishes a novel, *Trilby*, whose antihero Svengali has influenced generations about the nature of hypnosis.

Instead, without any of the mesmerists' hand passes, Braid simply got his subjects to focus on an object—usually the case in which he kept his lancet—and induced a trance. Braid also saw clearly that the power of the mind could affect the body, and he distinguished between different levels of trance.

However, though Braid was a respected physician, his views on hypnosis were not immediately accepted in the English-speaking world, in part because of the general mistrust of mesmerism. Instead, his ideas were to influence developments later in the nineteenth century in countries such as France.

American Pioneers

The European-born idea of mesmerism enjoyed a brief boom in the United States in the 1830s and 1840s. A number of European mesmerists, notably the Frenchman Charles Poyen St. Sauveur, introduced mesmerism to the United States in the 1830s and interest quickly grew. Soon the idea was being adapted by American practitioners who devised their own techniques and their own names for the phenomenon. One of the most famous American pioneers was La Roy Sunderland (1804–1885), who called the phenomenon "pathetism." His method was simply to talk about the subject to an audience until he had hypnotized a number of them. Another practitioner of mesmerism was Phineas Quimby (1802–1866), who discovered he could cure patients by putting *himself* in a trance and transferring "psychic energy" to the patient. Traveling road shows by mesmeric showmen were hugely popular. Ultimately, however, the interest in mesmerism and its various offshoots waned in the United States, as it had in Britain, as a revival in the churches and also in spiritism held sway.

Hypnosis—the Name

What we now know as hypnosis has been described by many different names during its history. Mesmer used the expression "animal magnetism," and his own name gave birth to the word "mesmerism" for those who followed his approach. In 1843 James Braid came up with the word "hypnotism," named for the Greek god of sleep, Hypnos, to describe the process. But even Braid doubted this was the right name, because he realized hypnosis did not involve sleep, and he later preferred the term "monoideism." One of his followers even described the process as "braidism" in honor of the Scottish physician, but that did not last, either. In the United States, terms such as "phrenomagnetism," "phrenomesmerism," and "electrobiology" were also used to describe essentially the same phenomenon.

Another name, used by the American La Roy Sunderland, was "pathetism," though he later abandoned this in favor of "electrical psychology." The multitude of different names demonstrates the confusion that existed among the early pioneers about what hypnosis was and how it worked.

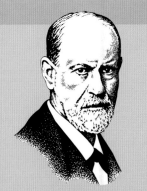

⤸The man who came up with the word "hypnosis" to describe the phenomenon—James Braid—later realized that its associations with the Greek god of sleep Hypnos were not helpful. But it was too late—the name had stuck.

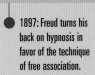

1900

1910

1897: Freud turns his back on hypnosis in favor of the technique of free association.

1913: Ormond McGill, one of the great American hypnotists of the twentieth century, is born in Palo Alto, California.

The French connection

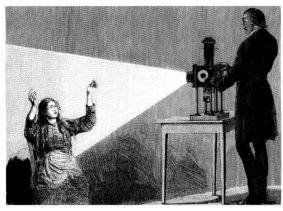

Interest in hypnosis in the United States and Britain declined during the middle of the nineteenth century, and it was left to France to lead the way. This was helped by two chance events. The first came in 1860, when a paper written by the Scottish pioneer of hypnosis James Braid was read at a scientific gathering in Paris. Among those present was a relatively obscure doctor by the name of Ambroise-Auguste Liébeault (1823–1904). Liébeault decided to try out the hypnotic techniques described in Braid's work and found that they were effective. In fact, the rural doctor

↶One of the ways scientists tried to explore the effects and depths of hypnosis was to see the effects of outside stimuli—such as light and darkness—on patients who were in a trance.

discovered that he did not even need to get the patient to stare at an object, as Braid had recommended. Simply by suggesting a trance, or a kind of sleep, as Liébeault believed it was, the doctor could induce it and use the power of suggestion to cure patients. This approach to hypnosis is quite similar to the modern one. However, the doctor lived in a small village near Nancy, northeast of Paris, and was working in near total obscurity. To make his discoveries known, Liébeault decided to publish a book of his findings. Yet this book sold no more than five copies in as many years, and it seemed as if Liébeault's contribution to hypnosis would remain in obscurity.

Then the second event occurred. A prominent professor of medicine at the University of Nancy had come to hear about Liébeault's ideas and was intrigued. The professor was Hippolyte Bernheim (1840–1919), who had sent an "incurable" patient to Liébeault. Bernheim's original aim had been to show up Liébeault as a fraud. Instead, he was so impressed with the physician's ability to cure the man's sciatica that he invited him to work with him at the university. Together, the two men founded what is known as the "Nancy school" of hypnosis. They believed hypnosis was psychological rather than physical and placed great emphasis on the importance of the power of suggestion. Bernheim and Liébeault also believed in establishing a rapport between doctor and patient, something many modern hypnotists consider important too. The fact that so eminent a man as Professor Bernheim was working with hypnosis helped secure it increased respectability.

1910

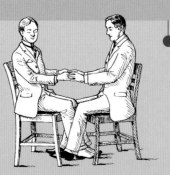

1914: World War I commences. There is renewed interest in hypnosis, owing to the number of paralytic and amnesia cases with psychogenic origin, and a scarcity of psychiatrists available.

1919: The French expert Pierre Janet published a book predicting the re-emergence of hypnosis.

1920

1923: Milton Erickson attends a lecture by the academic Clark Hull on hypnosis at Wisconsin University, and embarks on a journey to become America's most distinguished hypnotist.

Jean-Martin Charcot

Even more important, though, was the adoption of hypnosis by the most famous medical man of the day—Jean-Martin Charcot (1825–1904). Paris-based Charcot was an immensely talented scientist and physician who specialized in neurology. The charismatic Frenchman—his nickname was the "Napoléon of the neuroses"—was intrigued by hypnosis and used it on his patients. This move practically guaranteed that the subject would become accepted as a topic for serious research. The problem was that Charcot's views of hypnosis were at odds with those of the Nancy school and with most modern thinking on the issue. He believed that hypnosis was a form of hysteria, and that in some circumstances its use in therapy could even be dangerous. The two camps—Bernheim and Liébeault in Nancy, Charcot in Paris—quarreled bitterly about the true nature of hypnosis. Eventually, and for all Charcot's brilliance, the Nancy school of thought began to prevail and its influence was to last into the twentieth century. Hypnosis was becoming accepted as a subject of debate and research, but, unbeknownst to all of them, one of Charcot's former pupils was about to push hypnosis back into the scientific shadows.

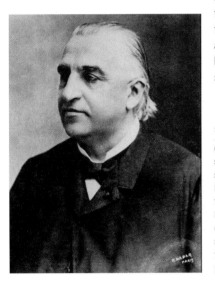

)Jean-Martin Charcot (1825–1904) was a gifted scientist and champion of studies into hypnosis. Dubbed the "Napoléon of the neuroses," Charcot became involved in a bitter dispute with a rival French school of scientists over the exact nature of the phenomenon.

The Automaton Argument

One of the areas in which the Nancy and Paris schools differed over hypnosis was the question of whether people could be persuaded to do anything against their will while in a trance. Bernheim argued that the hypnotic subject could effectively become an automaton, obedient to the will of the hypnotist. In one experiment, Bernheim hypnotized a male subject and told him that there was another man in the room who had insulted him. He suggested the subject kill the man with a dagger, handing him a paper knife as the weapon. The subject proceeded to stab the imaginary victim, and, when asked in a trance what he had done and why he had done it, the subject said that Bernheim had told him to kill the other man. The Paris school insisted that people do not lose their personality in hypnosis and may indulge in playacting. In a similar experiment by one of Charcot's followers, a woman in a trance cheerfully "murdered" a number of imaginary people, but, when some medical students suggested she undress and take a bath, she refused.

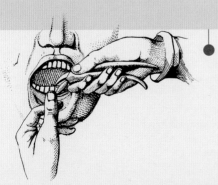

1925–47: Use of hypnosis in dentistry is developed in the United States.

1930s: The flamboyant American hypnotist Milton H. Erickson establishes his reputation as a leading authority on clinical hypnosis; he is a master of indirect hypnosis.

Freud and hypnosis

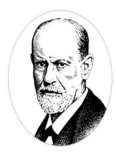

Sigmund Freud

Sigmund Freud (1856–1939) is well known as the most influential person in the history of psychology. Less well known is the fact that the father of psychoanalysis was a keen advocate of hypnosis early in his career. Indeed, it may be that Freud's later abandonment of it is one of the principal reasons why hypnosis languished in the scientific backwaters for much of the twentieth century, a position from which it is still gradually recovering.

The Austrian physician began his introduction to hypnosis in Paris in the 1880s under the tutelage of no less a figure than Jean-Martin Charcot, the leading French neurologist. In fact, Freud had been intrigued by the subject some years before, when, as a medical student in Vienna, he had watched a performance by the acclaimed Danish stage hypnotist Carl Hansen. What he saw in the show "firmly convinced me of the genuineness of the phenomenon of hypnosis," he later wrote.

For a number of years after his study under Charcot, Freud was a public advocate of hypnosis and used it in his own treatment. He used direct suggestion to the patients,

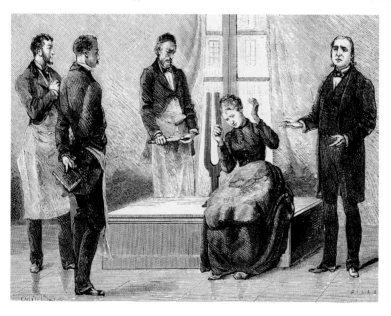

↵French scientist Jean-Martin Charcot is shown here demonstrating hypnosis to medical students with the aid of a tuning fork. One of the men who studied hypnosis under Charcot was Sigmund Freud, who was initially fascinated by the subject before rejecting it in favor of free association.

1930

1930: Clark Hull is forced to stop experiments using students because the authorities at Yale fear the dangers of hypnosis.

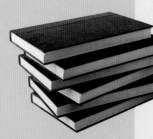

1940

1940s: Ormond McGill, one of the leading figures in hypnosis in the United States, starts publishing the first of more than thirty highly influential books on the subject.

occasionally pressing his hands on their heads as well. Freud also collaborated with his friend and fellow scientist Josef Breuer to use hypnotherapy on patients. Their best-known example was the case of a woman known as Anna O., who had a number of what were then called symptoms of hysteria. Breuer found that, when she was in a hypnotic trance, Anna was able to trace the association of these symptoms to real events in her life, and that by doing this she could apparently be cured of them. (It was later suggested, incidentally, that Anna had not been cured.)

Freud was fascinated by the hidden parts of the mind—the subconscious mind—and what impact they had on a person. The theories around hypnosis helped him to explore these ideas. However, by the mid-1890s he had abandoned hypnosis and instead developed his technique of free association, sometimes known as the "talking cure."

There is little doubt that Freud's decision was a blow for the future development of hypnosis. The Austrian went on to become the most influential voice of the twentieth century and inevitably, perhaps, his followers saw no reason to use hypnosis if the great man himself had discarded it.

It is important therefore to consider just why this brilliant man moved away from hypnosis into other areas. It was certainly not because he did not think it could work. Freud had been successful enough at the technique to know of its power. However, he felt that the suggestions used in hypnosis did not have a lasting effect, and he was also worried that patients would become too dependent on therapists by transferring their intense emotions onto them in a process called transference.

Some critics have suggested that Freud was simply not very good at hypnosis and so came up with a new technique—free association—that he was good at. More plausibly, perhaps, Freud was not happy with the authoritarian way in which hypnosis was usually carried out at that time. Patients were told they were going into sleep in a very direct way, which contrasts with the indirect, or so-called permissive, techniques favored today.

Whatever the real reasons, Freud's departure from the scene made it hard for hypnosis to establish itself at the forefront of the science of the mind as the twentieth century dawned.

Freud as a Hypnotist

It is sometimes claimed that Freud had problems as a hypnotist because of his teeth. He had to wear dentures, and the unkind suggestion has been made that these were ill-fitting, making it difficult for him to give clear voice to his hypnotic suggestions. In his early days, though, Freud reported that he had been genuinely flattered by the gratitude of some of his patients for curing them during hypnosis. Sometimes, however, he was worried that his patents might be becoming too familiar. On one occasion Freud was deeply embarrassed when a woman patient wrapped her arms around him. Freud not only used hypnosis in his medical practice, he also gave lectures and wrote studies on the subject. He even translated a book by the leading French hypnosis theoretician Hippolyte Bernheim.

1950

1943: The psychology professor George Estabrooks published a book claiming that hypnosis could have military uses.

1950s: The CIA experiments with hypnosis to interrogate spies and program agents.

1950: The word "brainwashing" is first used.

1951: A documented case in Sussex, England, in which Dr. A. Mason uses hypnotherapy to cure a teenage boy of the skin disease ichthyosis, helps gain acceptance for the medical role of hypnosis.

Twentieth-century hypnosis

By the start of the twentieth century, scientific interest in hypnosis was in decline, thanks in part to the new direction being forged by Sigmund Freud and others in psychoanalysis. Hypnosis was largely disregarded both as a tool to understand the mind, and as a method of therapy to cure patients. Not for the first time in its history, hypnosis became the province of the showmen and performers who wowed popular audiences while science looked disdainfully away. Even today, stage hypnotists claim it was their forebears who kept hypnosis alive and in the public domain during the years of the late nineteenth and early twentieth centuries.

⟨By the start of the twentieth century, and thanks to the rejection of hypnosis by the influential Sigmund Freud, most scientists dismissed the subject as unimportant. Apart from the efforts of a few lone medical experts, the art of hypnosis was largely kept alive in the public imagination by showmen and stage performers, and in popular fiction.

There were some experts, however, who continued to champion the cause of hypnosis. One was the Frenchman Pierre Janet (1859–1947). Janet came to believe that what he termed the subconscious was a permanent state that coexisted with the conscious. In hypnosis, Janet argued, the mind experienced dissociation, that is, was split between the conscious and subconscious. In a deep trance, this latter mind effectively took control. Janet's theories on the subconscious, and the notion that a person's problems could be forced back into his or her subconscious, where they could create hysterical symptoms, were similar to those of Freud. However, unlike his contemporary, Janet still believed in the usefulness of hypnosis. In 1919 he gloomily accepted that the subject was neglected, but predicted correctly that it would one day become a serious area of study again.

The terms "subconscious" and "unconscious," incidentally, are often used interchangeably, though they come from different analytical approaches. Generally, the subconscious comes from the tradition of Sigmund Freud, and the unconscious from his former collaborator Carl Gustav Jung (1875–1961).

Clark Hull

Another expert who maintained an interest in hypnosis was the American psychologist Boris Sidis, author of the influential book, *The Psychology of Suggestion* in 1898. In Britain, John Milne Bramwell's 1903 book, *Hypnotism: Its History, Practice and Theory*, also helped in keeping a flicker of academic interest alive.

1950

1952: The Hypnotism Act is passed in the U.K. to license stage hypnotists.

1955: The British Medical Association recognizes the benefits of hypnosis as a treatment for some ailments and in the relief of pain.

1958: The American Medical Association officially accepts the usefulness of hypnosis as a form of therapy.

1960

1962: The movie *The Manchurian Candidate* is released, highlighting fears of brainwashing.

Perhaps the major figure in hypnosis at this time was the American academic Clark Hull, one of the most respected psychologists of his generation. In 1918 Hull obtained a Ph.D. in psychology from the University of Wisconsin and for the next 15 years or so devoted much of his time to the study of hypnosis and in particular suggestibility. The result of these labors was his 1933 book, *Hypnosis and Suggestibility*, which has remained an important work on the subject. One of Hull's chief achievements was to encourage the use of hypnosis research at universities and other research institutes. Previously, much of the research had been carried out on patients by individual therapists, a process that often lacked scientific rigor. The scientific establishment was still however skeptical. In 1930 Hull, by now at Yale, was stopped from carrying out further hypnotic experiments on students because the authorities feared it was dangerous.

Apart from his own researches, Hull has another claim to prominence in the history of hypnosis: he excited the interest of a student who was to become the best-known hypnotist of the twentieth century.

Milton Erickson

During a lecture one day in 1923, a young psychology student at the University of Wisconsin was so fascinated by Clark Hull's demonstration of hypnosis that he later took the hypnotized person to one side to try out the procedure himself. It worked. That student was Milton Erickson (1901–1980) and from that time on he was set on the path to becoming the leading voice of hypnosis in America. He was both a researcher and a practitioner, who during his long career hypnotized many thousands of people. Erickson, who came from a poor background and suffered ill health most of his life, was an extraordinary, charismatic man, who put his emphasis on hypnosis as a therapeutic tool. One of his most important claims was that the unconscious mind is an immensely powerful tool for self-healing. Within each of us, Erickson believed, is the ability to help and heal ourselves.

Erickson's Personal Battle

Milton Erickson (pictured below) overcame a number of personal battles on his way to becoming America's most distinguished hypnotist. He was born in Nevada to a poor family. At the age of 17, Erickson contracted polio, which severely curtailed his movements, though he defied the doctors who said he would never walk again. Later in life, Erickson was to suffer an attack from another, different strain of polio and he once more fought back, though he spent the end of his life in a wheelchair. He said that the confining experience of polio as a young man had made him very aware of physical movement, and of how people communicated both verbally and nonverbally, which helped him in observing and understanding the reactions of patients. In addition, Erickson was both color-blind and tone-deaf. Nor were all his problems physical. Early in his career the medical authorities, who at the time distrusted hypnosis, threatened to remove his medical license. An amusing, though apocryphal, story has it that he hypnotized the members of the American Medical Association who were hearing his case to persuade them to let him keep his license.

1970   1980

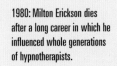

1980: Milton Erickson dies after a long career in which he influenced whole generations of hypnotherapists.

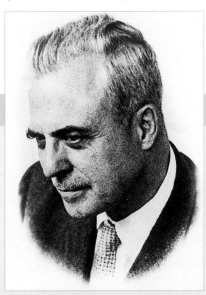

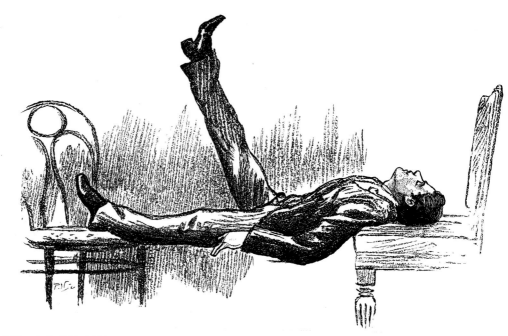

↪The American Milton Erickson was one of the men who realized the power of the unconscious mind and that hypnosis could be used to influence it. His charisma and success with the technique helped give hypnosis back renewed credibility and popularity during the twentieth century.

Perhaps his biggest contribution to hypnosis was his development of powerful new techniques of inducing a trance and imparting suggestions to the unconscious mind. Previous methods of trance induction had tended to be quite authoritarian and dogmatic: the patients were told they were feeling sleepy and going into a trance. Erickson did not reject this approach completely, but believed in adapting the therapist's technique according to the individual patient's character and needs. He developed what are known as indirect or "permissive" techniques, in which, through the use of language, the patients would become part of a two-way process. They effectively put themselves into a trance. One famous technique was that of "confusion," where, by the use of meaningless words in jumbled-up sentences, the conscious mind would become distracted, and the patient would go into a trance. Erickson also developed the use of metaphors and storytelling in hypnosis; for him, the imaginative use of language was very important. He was always creative in his approach to patients and believed that just about anyone could be hypnotized; it depended on the skill and flexibility of the hypnotist. Though Erickson wrote widely on hypnosis, it is this practical and creative approach to hypnotherapy that has become his lasting legacy. Many current practitioners have been inspired by his work.

1990

1993: A British woman, Sharron Tabarn, dies following a seizure that occurs five hours after she took part as a volunteer in a stage hypnosis show.

1993: The American Psychiatric Association warns that memories recovered in therapy, including hypnosis, could be false.

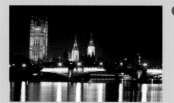

1994: The case of Ms. Tabarn and other incidents of hypnotism are debated in the British Parliament. The government promises a review of the 1952 Hypnotism Act.

The Hypnosis Debate

Another very influential American hypnotherapist was Dave Elman (1900–1967), the son of a stage hypnotist, who developed very rapid and effective trance-induction techniques. Elman placed great emphasis on the need to be able to bypass the mind's critical faculty in order for a person to go into a trance. As with Milton Erickson, his techniques and approach to hypnosis are widely followed among therapists who are working today.

By the second half of the twentieth century the therapeutic use of hypnosis—hypnotherapy—was on the increase. Meanwhile, two different and conflicting theories of the nature of hypnosis were also developing.

On one side of the argument were those who believed that a person enters an altered state of consciousness during hypnosis. On the other side were the academics who claim that there is no such thing as a hypnotic state and that everything that happens in hypnosis can be explained by existing psychological phenomena—otherwise known as the nonstate school of thought. In the latter school of thought there have been American academics, such as Theodore Xenophon Barber, who argue that what occurs to a patient during hypnosis results from "task motivation," that is, the desire to do what is required and needed of them. He also argues that what occurs is an act of the patient's imagination.

Against this there are theorists such as the late Ernest Hilgard, a long-time professor of psychology at Stanford and a pioneer of the scientific study of hypnosis in the second half of the twentieth century. Hilgard's view was that there are behaviors that are unique to people who are hypnotized. He avoided the word "state" but instead referred to a "domain of hypnosis." The debate about the very nature of hypnosis rages on to this day (see page 38).

George Estabrooks

Another influential figure in twentieth-century hypnosis, but a contrasting character to Milton Erickson, was the professor of psychology at Colgate University, George Estabrooks (1895–1973). Estabrooks was a proponent of the traditional, direct approach to trance induction in hypnosis. Typically, this means saying to the patient phrases such as, "... You are falling asleep ... you will not wake up till I tell you ..." He was also convinced of the potential use—and abuse—of hypnosis in warfare and espionage. He declared, "I can hypnotize a man without his knowledge or consent into committing treason against the United States."

In his 1943 book, *Hypnotism*, Estabrooks suggested that squads of hypnotized enemy agents could cause havoc to America's defenses. Two years later, Estabrooks helped write a novel called *Death in the Mind*, in which the Germans managed to hypnotize American servicemen into sabotaging their own side.

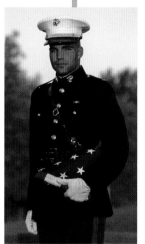

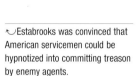
⌒Estabrooks was convinced that American servicemen could be hypnotized into committing treason by enemy agents.

2000

1995: A panel of experts convened by the British Government rules that there is no evidence of serious risk to participants in stage hypnosis. However, certain licensing laws in the 1952 Act are tightened.

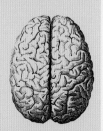

2001: Results of a Harvard University study indicate that brain activity does change in people under hypnosis; it backs the argument that there is a specific state of hypnosis.

The state of hypnosis today

At the start of the twenty-first century, the story of hypnosis has come a long way. From its unpromising origins in Franz Anton Mesmer's animal magnetism, hypnosis is now established as a legitimate field of scientific research and as a valuable therapeutic tool. Each day tens of thousands of people in America, Europe, and the rest of the world use hypnosis to help remove a bad habit, ease pain, or perform some other kind of therapy. Sports performers, statesmen, media stars, and top businesspeople are known to have used the technique to enhance their lives. And yet the subject is still viewed with mistrust by a large number of ordinary people. The old fears associated with hypnosis in the past—that it was somehow connected with the occult, or was simply a fraud or just for entertainment—linger on. In part, this is due to the way that hypnosis has been portrayed in society through various forms of media. In part, too, we can blame some users of hypnosis at the fringe of the debate who have put the technique to dubious purposes, such as learning how to hypnotize members of the opposite sex. These tacky uses have simply confirmed people's worst prejudices about the subject.

Another reason for some people's reluctance to take hypnosis seriously is that scientists still cannot adequately explain how it works. While academics continue to debate the true nature of hypnosis, or whether it is even "real," the public can perhaps be forgiven for viewing it with bewilderment.

⸔Hypnosis is widely used today not just in medicine but also by top sports performers, business experts, and those in the media to boost their performance and mental focus. Despite this, many members of the public still view hypnosis with fear and suspicion.

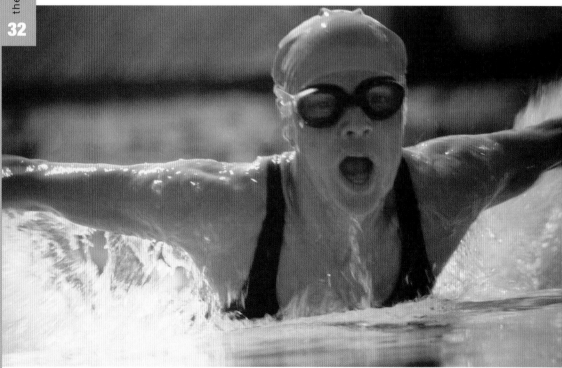

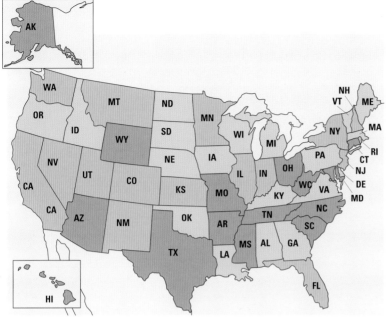

Safe Practice States

Guild Standard States

Regulated States

The good news is that hypnosis is steadily gaining acceptance in the medical world. As long ago as 1958 the American Medical Association declared that it was a safe practice with no harmful side effects. Three years previously, the British Medical Association had similarly endorsed hypnosis as a useful therapeutic tool in the treatment of some psychoneuroses and also in pain relief. Meanwhile, a number of hospitals, in America and elsewhere, are beginning to use hypnosis in pain relief and in helping patients come to terms with other forms of treatment such as chemotherapy.

The situation with hypnotherapists and clinical hypnotists who deal directly with the public is more confused. A bewildering number of different training and accreditation organizations have been set up in recent decades. The classic model is for a new association to establish its own school, and then recognize that school's qualifications. Some of these organizations have good track records in training therapists; others are less impressive. The problem here is the lack of legal checks, although some states in America now have legislation that controls medical uses of hypnosis through a license system. A license on its own, of course, is no guarantee of quality unless it is backed by strict training criteria and proper administrative overseeing. In any case, some of the best practitioners are "lay hypnotists," who come from a long tradition and who may have little formal training. Some of the best therapeutic hypnotists are also stage performers, who may or may not possess recognized medical qualifications.

The legal situation regarding hypnotists and therapy could certainly be clarified and improved. Equally important, though, is that research should continue into the phenomenon itself, a process that has been only fitful in the past. Society will be far more open to the idea of hypnotism when we gain a fuller understanding of its real nature.

◡Unlike much of the rest of the world, some states in America have introduced legislation that controls medical uses of hypnosis through a license system. An important distinction exists between "certified" and "licensed" practitioners. The former will be trained in hypnosis but not (necessarily) medically trained. The latter should have credentials in healthcare as well as in hypnosis. In the United States, the only two nationally recognized organizations for licensed healthcare professionals using hypnosis are the Society for Clinical and Experimental Hypnosis and the American Society of Clinical Hypnosis. When seeking mental health therapy, it is important that patients look for licensed professionals.

Safe Practice States: You may freely practice in accordance with the recommended Standards of the Guild.

Guild Standard States: There are one or more laws that prohibit a Guild hypnotist who is not otherwise qualified to practice some other profession from practicing hypnotism.

Regulated States: There is a specific law in these states that regulates the practice of hypnotism.

Hypnosis in the media

The bad image of hypnosis at the end of the twentieth century was partly because of the way it was portrayed by journalists and writers. In particular novelist George du Maurier created the malevolent character of a hypnotist called Svengali in his novel *Trilby*. Ever since, the word Svengali has been associated with men who try to bring unwilling female victims under their control—an inaccurate description of how hypnosis works.

The way in which society sees hypnosis is influenced by the way the media portray it. With some exceptions, that portrayal has been negative. A classic depiction of hypnosis was given in the 1962 movie *The Manchurian Candidate,* a Cold War thriller that warned of the dangers of brainwashing. While *The Manchurian Candidate* is a very good film, its depiction of hypnosis is misleading; and other movies, books, and television programs have been simply sensationalist.

Svengali

If a single person must be blamed for the popular image of hypnosis, then that person would probably be the British illustrator and writer George du Maurier (1834–1896). In 1894 he published *Trilby,* which introduced a name still common in the English language—Svengali. The word is now defined by *The Chambers Dictionary* as "a person who exerts total mental control over another, usually for evil ends." In the novel, Svengali uses hypnosis to control the heroine, the young artist's model Trilby O'Ferrall. The mysterious, bearded Hungarian with staring eyes turns Trilby into an acclaimed singer, becoming her manager and her husband. When Svengali dies, Trilby's singing powers end also, as she is able to perform only under the influence of his powerful gaze.

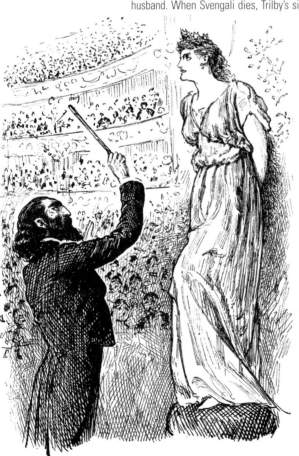

Trilby was a best-seller and gave to the world the idea that hypnosis could be misused. Even today, the image of a bearded man with staring eyes is not far away from many people's idea of hypnosis. *Trilby* left the public with two lasting impressions about hypnosis. The first was that someone can be kept in a trance, and the second was that a person can be made to do something under hypnosis that he or she would not usually do. Interestingly, in the 1840s the hypnosis pioneer James Braid had himself helped a young woman sing to an ability far beyond her earlier efforts, though whether du Maurier knew of that case is unclear.

Other Fiction

Other well-known writers who have portrayed hypnosis include Sir Arthur Conan Doyle in his short story *The Great Keinplatz Experiment,* Edgar Allen Poe in *The Facts in the Case of M. Valdemar,* and Thomas Mann in his novel *Mario and the Magician.* None of these are very positive portrayals of the technique.

Movies

Hollywood has made good use of the dramatic possibilities of hypnosis, in addition to *The Manchurian Candidate*. One good example was the 1949 movie *Whirlpool,* in which a hypnotist hypnotizes a woman into helping him to blackmail her husband. In *Rasputin: The Mad Monk* (1966), the Russian is portrayed as a Svengali-like character with staring eyes and a long beard, who hypnotizes the tsar and his family. There is in fact no evidence that Rasputin used hypnosis, until possibly a few months before his death when he reportedly took lessons in the technique in a vain attempt to revive what he considered to be his flagging influence.

More recently, hypnosis played a central role in the plot of Woody Allen's 2001 movie *The Curse of the Jade Scorpion.* An unscrupulous hypnotist turns an insurance investigator into a jewel thief and causes him to fall in love with a woman he can't stand. It is an amusing but not very flattering view of hypnosis.

Television

The use of hypnosis has become a regular feature of many television programs. The list of shows that have used hypnosis as part of a plot includes "Batman," "Lost in Space," "The Avengers," "The Man from U.N.C.L.E.," "Star Trek," "Superman," "Columbo," "Charlie's Angels," "General Hospital," "Beverley Hills 90210," and "Voyage to the Bottom of the Sea." Although much of the time hypnosis has been portrayed as something strange or threatening, there have been examples of a more considered and knowledgeable approach. In "The X Files" series, for example, FBI agent Fox Mulder uses hypnosis, including age regression, in an attempt to recall what happened to his missing sister. In one episode Mulder even refers to the ability of Franz Anton Mesmer, the eighteenth-century proponent of mesmerism, to hypnotize an entire audience. Hypnosis is treated in a calm, sober manner that reflects its uses as well as potential abuses.

Other Media

Newspapers and magazines have varied widely in their coverage of hypnosis. The more excitable publications have tended to focus on lurid claims of staring-eyed characters seducing women, or therapists abusing patients. Gradually, however, the more serious newspapers and magazines around the world have begun to run more considered articles on the subject, as scientific research has confirmed the usefulness of hypnosis in therapeutic settings.

The Fu Manchu Books and Movies

One of the most notorious depictions of hypnosis as malevolent has been in the Fu Manchu films, based on the novels of Sax Rohmer. Just about the only person able to resist Fu Manchu's hypnotic stare is, it seems, the British policeman Sir Dennis Nayland Smith of Scotland Yard. In *The Brides of Fu Manchu* (1966), Fu Manchu hypnotizes a young woman who then, apparently unaware of what she is doing, kills another woman. The daughter of Fu Manchu is also shown to be able to control people's actions through hypnosis. All of this is good entertainment even if it is totally misleading about the power of hypnosis.

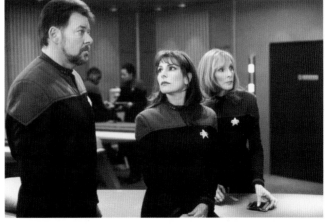

The portrayal of hypnotized people in television shows (as shown below in a scene from "Star Trek") or in movies can be misleading. Unfortunately the public is influenced by what it sees.

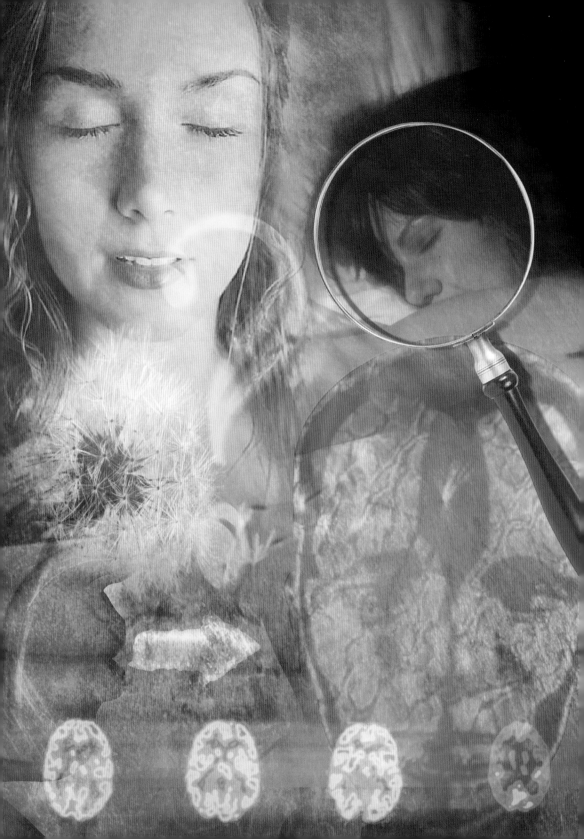

2: The Nature of Hypnosis

How hypnosis works—and what it is—has long baffled scientists. Even today, when our understanding of the human brain and mind has increased so dramatically, the precise nature of hypnosis is still disputed. What seems clear, however, is that the phenomenon of hypnosis is real and measurable. The inducing of a trance, the power of suggestion, and the lasting effects have all been examined by scientists. Ultimately, the nature of hypnosis is intimately linked with the subtle relationship between different states of our mind—the conscious and the unconscious.

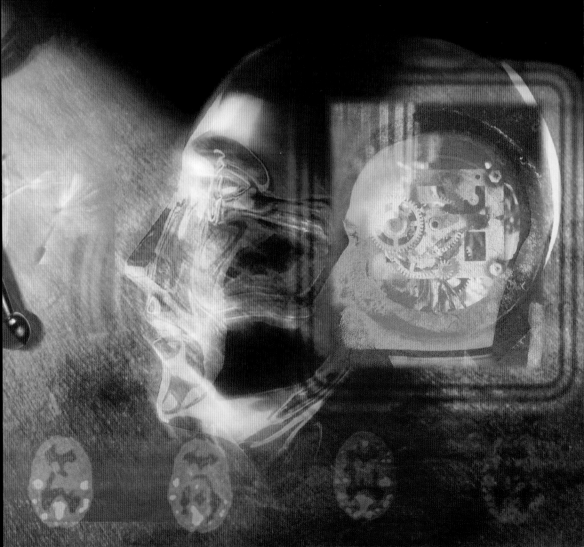

What is hypnotism?

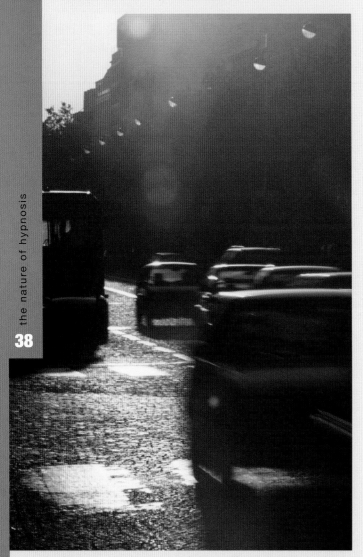

Despite the many startling advances of modern science, the subtle and elaborate workings of the human mind are still not fully understood. It should therefore come as no surprise to learn that academics disagree about what hypnosis is, and how it works. This does not mean that it is not real; in fact, scientists have demonstrated in recent experiments that people's brains do undergo changes when they have been hypnotized (see page 39). Moreover, many medical experts accept that hypnosis can be a powerful tool in the treatment of some conditions and also in the alleviation of pain. However, there is as yet no universally accepted theory to explain exactly what hypnosis is and how it works, and there exist a number of different and in some cases conflicting scientific views.

The first point to make is that, despite the origin of its name, hypnosis does not involve sleep. When a person is in a hypnotic trance, the body may be in a very relaxed state, but the mind is alert and highly focused. It is also a very natural state. All of us experience a trancelike state many times in our daily lives. Those of us who drive cars are very familiar with the phenomenon of driving along a well-known route and arriving at our destination—and then being aware that we can't remember the journey at all. It is as if we were on autopilot for the journey, and in a sense we were. We were in a kind of trance.

⤸No one yet fully understands how hypnosis works; but we know that during a trance our bodies are very relaxed while our minds are very focused. It has been likened to that feeling we experience when we drive for miles to a familiar destination without being consciously aware of the process of driving.

The same can occur when we are engrossed in a movie, reading a book, listening to music, or gazing into the eyes of someone we love. Time seems to stand still and we are oblivious of the outside world, our attention completely focused on what we are doing at that moment. That, too, can be described as a trance. Many people also consider a trance to be the state achieved in meditation or when we are daydreaming. These examples are not hypnotic trances, but they do demonstrate how our conscious minds can become distracted as we become absorbed in a particular activity.

Hypnotic Trance

The hypnotic trance, then, is an essential element of hypnosis. A key difference between the sorts of trance described earlier and the hypnotic trance is that during the latter there is another person—the hypnotist—who is guiding us into this state. Hypnosis alone is simply a state of mind, and bringing it about is simply a technique. The process of helping someone into a hypnotic trance is called induction. Techniques of induction can vary widely, and have progressed from the clichéd method of swinging a watch in front of the patient's eyes. Before trance induction begins, the therapeutic hypnotist generally spends time with the subject, assessing his or her personality, likes, dislikes, and aims. The therapist will also try to discover how open that person is to being put into a hypnotic trance.

On its own, a hypnotic trance does not do anything except alter our state of mind. This is sometimes referred to as neutral hypnosis. For us to change our behavior— whether giving up smoking or quitting drinking—we need to be reprogrammed. This is where the work of a clinical hypnotist or a hypnotherapist differs from that of a stage hypnotist. While stage hypnotists use hypnosis for entertainment, hypnotherapists use it to help people get better. To do this the hypnotist needs to make suggestions to the subject. These suggestions are the triggers that aim to change people's habits, boost their confidence, or help them come to terms with their past. Such suggestions are made not to our conscious mind, but to our unconscious mind, the part of the mind that controls so much of our lives.

↪There is now scientific proof that our brains do alter during a hypnotic trance; scientists at Harvard University found evidence of changes in the brain using positron-emission tomography (PET) scanners.

Brain Research

A fascinating experiment by researchers at Harvard University has produced evidence that the brain does behave differently when a person is under hypnosis. These findings back up the theory that there is an altered state of consciousness known as a hypnotic state. The research team, which included Stephen Kosslyn, professor of psychology at Harvard, and David Spiegel of Stanford University School of Medicine, hypnotized eight people and monitored their brains with a positron-emission tomography (PET) scanner. The subjects were then shown brightly colored shapes and told to imagine they were gray, and then shown gray shapes and told to imagine they were colored. The experiment was also done while the subjects were not hypnotized. The researchers discovered that, when not hypnotized, the subjects showed a change in brain activity only in their right hemisphere while they were imagining the change of color. But, when they were under hypnosis, the left hemisphere also showed a change of activity, as well as the right. The findings suggest that a genuine change occurs in our brains during a hypnotic trance.

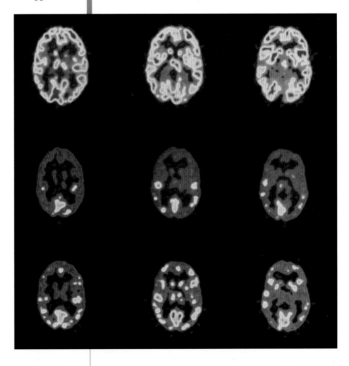

The unconscious mind

To understand the basis of hypnosis, it is important to grasp the distinction between the conscious and unconscious minds (see page 41). We actively think and take part in life through the conscious mind, which uses reason and logic, and solves problems. It is governed by the left side of the brain, which is predominantly verbal in the way it works.

The unconscious mind, governed by our right brain, which is predominantly visual, regulates our autonomic nervous system, which in turn governs the involuntary functions of the body, keeping the heart pumping, the blood circulating, and the lungs breathing. The unconscious mind is also the repository of all our thoughts, memories, and emotions. It is constantly aware of all our sensations and thoughts, although the conscious mind is aware of only a tiny fraction of these.

The unconscious mind is where our habits and behavioral patterns reside. We are not always aware of why we react as we do to certain events; we just know that we react. It is the unconscious mind that governs those reactions, based on the information and emotions it has stored. The unconscious mind maintains our view of reality and houses the experiences that, along with our genes, determine our personalities.

Reprogramming

Our conscious minds are dimly aware of the existence of the other mind. Most people are familiar with what happens when we "sleep on" a problem. If we forget about the matter and go to sleep, we often find that when we wake up in the morning we have a solution. This is the work of the unconscious mind, sifting through ideas until it comes up with an answer. This small example gives some glimpse of the potential power of the unconscious mind.

The unconscious mind could be regarded as a computer, operating programs that it has built over years from past experiences, thoughts, and emotions. Sometimes these programs are useful for assisting our conscious aims; sometimes they are not. For example, one person might feel perfectly confident about speaking in public, whereas another may develop a nervous rash at the thought of having to do so, even though rationally there may be nothing to worry about. In this example, their unconscious minds may simply be running different programs.

To reprogram the mind, the hypnotist must communicate

The Conscious Mind	The Unconscious Mind
Analytic	Intuitive, imaginative
Verbal	Spatial
Rational	Synthetic
Logical	Creative
Sequential, linear	Simultaneous, holistic
Time-orientated	Timeless, spiritual
Scientific	Musical
Mathematic	Artistic
Frank, direct	Flexible
Sensible	Playful, fanciful
Forceful	Complex

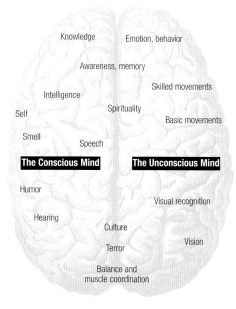

Knowledge
Emotion, behavior
Awareness, memory
Skilled movements
Intelligence
Self
Spirituality
Basic movements
Smell
Speech
The Conscious Mind   **The Unconscious Mind**
Humor
Visual recognition
Hearing
Culture
Terror
Vision
Balance and muscle coordination

↪Scientists are beginning to discover more about how our brain and our mind works. The left-hand side of the brain is governed more by verbal stimuli and is the realm of logic; it is the seat of our conscious mind. The right-hand side is where our unconscious mind resides, which responds to visual stimuli and is the realm of our imagination.

directly with the unconscious mind. This does not mean that the hypnotist controls the unconscious mind or forcibly changes it. According to the late American professor of psychology Ernest Hilgard, no matter how deep the trance and how effective the hypnotist, there is always a part of the mind that knows what is going on—the "hidden observer." In one experiment, a woman was hypnotized and Hilgard induced anesthesia in one of her arms. She then put this arm into a bucket of iced water. When asked in the trance, she said she felt no pain. However, she had also been asked to write down with her other hand what pain she was experiencing. Her writing—a series of numbers on a scale of one to ten—indicated that she was aware of the pain, despite what she was saying. This led to the idea that a part of us is always aware even when we are in a different state of mind. Some experts suggest that this "hidden observer" is in fact our consciousness, always present even when we are in a deep trance.

In some fields of psychotherapy there is a process known as reframing, in which the patient is encouraged to see the world in a new way. In a sense, this is what the hypnotherapist is trying to do with the patient's unconscious mind. The unconscious mind works to its own reasoning based on associations built up over time. While, in the example given earlier, it may be illogical that a person should be terrified of public speaking, to the unconscious mind it makes sense based on past associations made with the act of public speaking. The hypnotherapist will build different, more positive associations so that the unconscious mind no longer links the activity with fear but with something good. A more general aim is to help people to become in tune with their unconscious minds, so that, instead of pulling in different directions, conscious and unconscious minds work together.

The terms "subconscious" and "unconscious" are often used interchangeably, though, confusingly, different experts and academic traditions have also used the terms to mean different concepts. For example, Sigmund Freud and his former collaborator Carl Gustav Jung used the terms in different contexts. For consistency, this book will normally use just one term: unconscious.

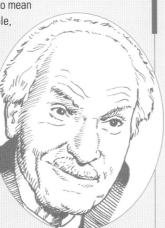

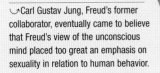
↪Carl Gustav Jung, Freud's former collaborator, eventually came to believe that Freud's view of the unconscious mind placed too great an emphasis on sexuality in relation to human behavior.

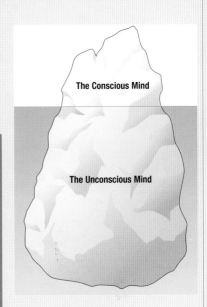

The Conscious Mind

The Unconscious Mind

It's All in the Mind

The distinction drawn between the conscious and unconscious should be regarded as no more than a useful model to help us understand the different functions of the mind. The conscious and unconscious minds are in reality not distinct entities, but are more accurately seen as a spectrum of one mind. According to this view, our mind displays various phenomena, which we find useful to categorize by the general terms conscious and unconscious. One image used to try to explain this sees the mind as an iceberg: the small amount showing above the water is the conscious, while the submerged part is the unconscious.

Another model sees the mind as a darkened room. If you shine a flashlight around the room you will illuminate certain details, which represent the conscious mind, while the unlit rest of the room is the unconscious mind. Both examples help us understand that the conscious and unconscious are both present at the same time.

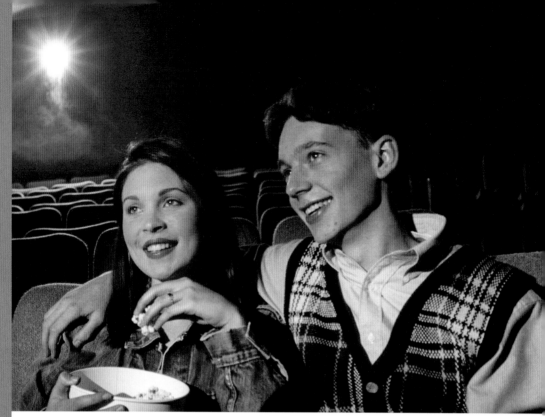

The theories of hypnotism

No one is sure how hypnosis works, and there is no one agreed definition about what hypnotism is. Hypnotists themselves concur on the essential element of hypnotism, that a person goes into a trance, but even here it is unclear just what is meant by this. They merely agree that it works. The most accepted view among practitioners is that patients enter an altered state of consciousness. In this altered state the hypnotist talks directly to the unconscious mind. The conscious mind, which possesses critical faculties and is therefore a potential barrier to this communication, is encouraged into the background.

One way of looking at this process is to consider how we view films, read novels, or watch plays at the theater. We know that the characters are not real and are just fictional creations by the author, yet we still react to them and their actions as if they were real. We are happy to laugh or cry with the characters or feel scared, for example, by scenes in horror movies, even though they are make-believe. This is commonly known as the suspension of disbelief. In a similar way, our unconscious has its own sense of what is real. For the unconscious, what is real is whatever it knows. This explains why a hypnotist who has put a person into a deep trance can make the subject believe that a sour lemon really tastes like a piece of candy or react to a fragrant rose as if it smelled like an old sock. It is the unconscious mind that is adopting these suggestions as new reality and the rest of the body, brain, and mind behave accordingly.

↶We all experience the working of our unconscious minds on a daily basis. When we are watching a movie, reading a novel, or seeing a play, part of us accepts the characters and scenes we see as "real" even though we know they are fictional creations; this is sometimes known as the suspension of disbelief.

The hypnotists' view of hypnotism is not universally accepted by all academics. Some consider that hypnotic subjects do not enter a trance, and dispute the physical reality of the altered state of consciousness. They argue that what we consider to be hypnosis is really the subject's reaction to personal beliefs and expectations, and the situation. This view of hypnosis suggests that people are in fact merely role-playing, with the subject playing the role of the hypnotized patient. We think and expect that the hypnotist will put us into a hypnotic trance, so this is what we think has happened to us. These critics point out that the behavior exhibited in hypnosis can be induced in people by other means. This approach to hypnosis has been challenged in recent years by those studies that show that the brains of people under hypnosis do exhibit subtle changes.

In any case, none of the academic disputes mean that hypnosis is not real. There are many areas in the scientific world where there are no universally accepted theories to explain observed phenomena. We may have considered how apples still fell to the ground before Isaac Newton came up with the theory of gravity.

The crucial point is that when a hypnotist makes suggestions to what we think of as a person's subconscious mind, while he or she is in a trancelike state, it works. A precise and widely accepted theory of how and why it works may have to wait for a later scientific advance.

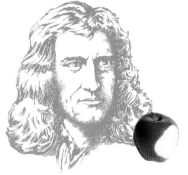

⌣While no one has yet come up with a complete theory to explain what hypnosis is and how it works, this does not mean it is not real. Apples still fell to the ground before Isaac Newton (pictured) put forward the theory of gravity.

Hypnotic Theories

There have been and remain many different theories to explain the phenomenon of hypnosis, stretching back to one of the leading figures in the history of hypnosis, the nineteenth-century Scotsman James Braid (see page 22), and to the founder of psychoanalysis and one-time champion of hypnosis, Sigmund Freud (see page 26). The Frenchman Pierre Janet, a contemporary of Freud, thought hypnosis occurred through "dissociation," a splitting off of part of the mind. The "conditioned-reflex" theory holds that people under hypnosis have been conditioned by the general—society's—view of hypnosis to show the expected reactions. Meanwhile, the role-playing theory suggests that the client or patient is assuming the role of the hypnotized person and does his or her best to play that part. The core difference is between those experts who consider that there is an altered state of consciousness (ASC) during the hypnosis process (the state theorists), and those who insist there is no different state and that all the phenomena of so-called hypnosis can be explained by existing psychological phenomena (the nonstate theorists).

⌣During a trance, the aim of the hypnotist is to talk directly to the patient's unconscious mind. The conscious mind can act as a barrier to this communication, and so is either distracted or encouraged to be still.

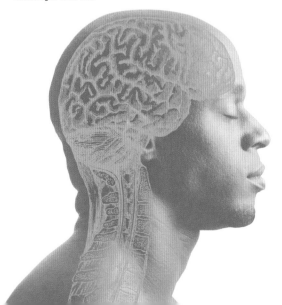

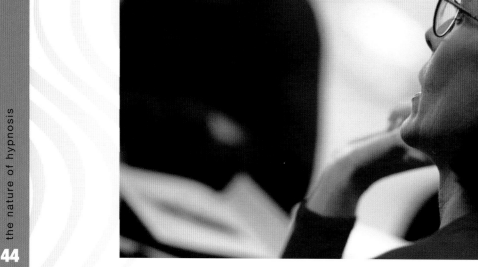

Before the trance

The relationship between the hypnotherapist and the subject is an important one. In the everyday trances that we experience, such as daydreaming or when we are watching television, we are in our own world with no one else. When someone is being guided into a trance by another person, then the hypnotist becomes the focus of the subject's unconscious mind and his or her role is crucial. It makes a difference if there is a high level of trust between the subject and the hypnotist. For many people the thought of going under hypnosis for the first time can be quite unnerving. We don't know what to expect or what is going to happen to us. When we put ourselves in the hands of someone who will take us beyond our conscious mind into the realm of the unconscious, we like to feel that we have total confidence in him or her.

A hypnotist will spend some time talking to the subject. The aim is to discover the person's interests, desires, fears, and aims for the session. This helps build up trust. If you do not feel comfortable with your hypnotist or do not feel that you can trust him or her, you should walk away.

The prehypnosis interview is also important for other reasons as well. From the information and personality of the subject, the hypnotist will work out how best to

↶Hypnotherapists will usually spend some time talking to their clients before putting them into a trance. It is important the hypnotist understands the real needs of the client, as well as his or her hopes and fears. This is also a chance for clients to discover if he or she feels comfortable with the hypnotist.

handle the session. The hypnotist needs to discover how skeptical subjects are about hypnosis and whether they believe they can be put into a trance. From this talk the hypnotist will also work out what words to use for the suggestions made during the trance—the script. Often the hypnotist and the patient will write this script together. This ensures that subjects feel confident they know what is going to be suggested to their unconscious minds, and are sure that it fits in with their aims, as well as their moral and ethical beliefs.

Another purpose of the pretrance talk is for the hypnotherapist to discover how open to hypnotic suggestion subjects are, and, more importantly, to convince them that they are suggestible. This is particularly important with clients who are skeptical about the whole process. Though anyone can potentially be put into a trance and be open to hypnotic suggestion, the more someone believes in it, the easier it will be and the more beneficial the process is likely to be.

These so-called suggestibility tests are simple but can be very effective. A common one is for the hypnotist to ask the subject to put both arms out straight in front at shoulder level. The person's eyes should be closed. The hypnotist then asks the patient to imagine that attached to one hand is a lighter-than-air object—it may be a helium-filled balloon—that is pulling that arm up. Meanwhile the client imagines that the other hand is attached to a heavy object, such as a book, or maybe a small bucket slowly filling with water. This is dragging that arm down.

If the client moves one or both arms even slightly, as subjects often do, then this reaction is used as proof of the power of the imagination. The conscious mind knows that neither balloon nor bucket is there, but the unconscious reacts to the suggestion that they are. By convincing clients that they are hypnotizable, the hypnotist has already begun the process of hypnosis. Stage hypnotists sometimes start their act by showing the audience someone they have hypnotized before the show. This gets the spectators to expect that hypnosis will take place during the show, which makes the task of hypnotizing much more straightforward.

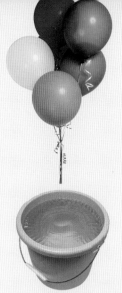

↶Often the hypnotist will ask the patient to take part in a test of his or her imagination. A common one is for the person to imagine that one arm is tied to helium-filled balloons, pulling that arm up, while the other is attached to a bucket slowly filling with water, pulling that arm down. These so-called suggestibility tests help the patient believe in the power of the imagination.

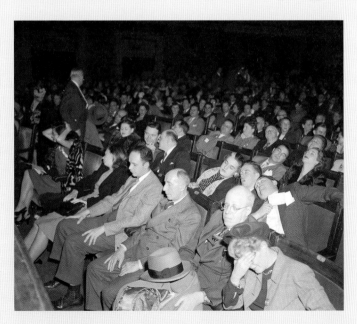

↶The process of hypnosis is much easier for the stage hypnotist if the audience is already expecting it to take place.

The trance state

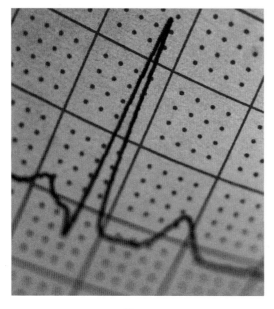

An important part of hypnosis is the trance state. It is here that the unconscious mind is freed from the critical fetters of the conscious mind and is open to suggestion.

First of all, let us consider the different states of mind that we experience. The first is usually experienced in our waking lives and is known as the beta state. In this state our brains are highly alert, and this is when reasoning and logic are employed. Scientists have measured the activity of our brains during different states, and can monitor the activity using an electroencephalograph (EEG). At beta state our brain waves vary between about 14 and 30 cycles per second (c.p.s.).

The second state of mind is called the alpha state, when our brain waves operate at between 8 and 13 c.p.s. In this state our minds are still alert but are more relaxed. We are generally more creative in this state of mind, more open to information and imagination. Some hypnotists see this state as the

⌣An electroencephalograph (EEG) is a machine that records electrical currents generated in our brains. Scientists and medical researchers can use these tests to measure the different levels of brain activity we exhibit according to what state our minds are in.

⌣Different wavelengths of electrical activity exist in our brains at any one time. According to which brain waves are predominant, our states of mind may be called alpha, beta, theta, or delta state. The beta state is associated with our normal, waking state.

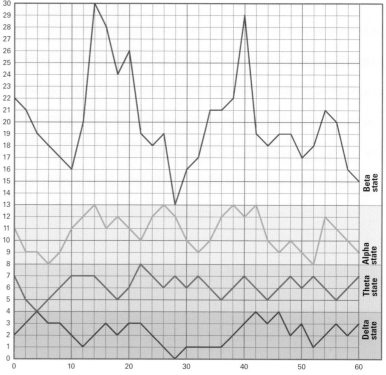

gateway from the conscious into the unconscious mind. The alpha state is an everyday experience for us, whether we are wrapped up in a movie or going into or out of sleep. Hypnotists say that when we enter the alpha state we are moving into a trance.

The third state is called theta, in which the brain waves are between 4 and 8 c.p.s. This state is associated with deep relaxation, tranquility, and dreams. Theta is sometimes known as the dream state. We pass through the theta state on the way to and from deep sleep.

The final state is called delta, when the brain waves are below 4 c.p.s. This is the deep-sleep state, where there is total unawareness from the mind, and it is not a state reached in hypnosis.

It should be pointed out that these levels of brain waves are not neatly restricted to one state of mind. For example, there are alpha waves or theta waves in our brains even when we are in the beta or waking state. The four stages refer to the occasions when those particular wavelengths predominate. The significance of these states for hypnosis is that it is during the alpha and theta states that the hypnotic trance exists. It is then that suggestions to the always-present unconscious mind are not obstructed by the critical faculties of the conscious mind. When the patient has begun to allay those critical faculties—the process of suspension of disbelief—then suggestions can be used to work on the unconscious.

The hypnotic trance is often divided into six different stages or depths, which occur in the alpha and theta states right down to the beginning of the delta state.

Each of these six stages is associated with different experiences that can be induced by the hypnotist. Hypnotists learn both how to induce these different levels of trance and how to identify them.

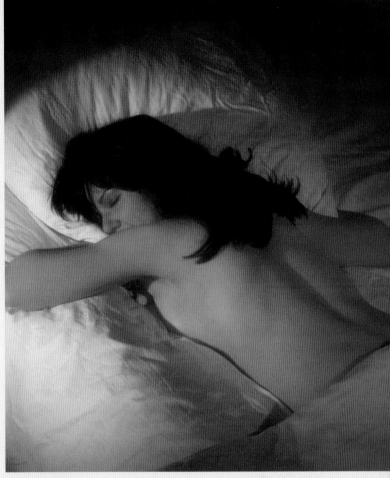

↳The delta state of mind is known as the deep-sleep state in which our brain waves are below four cycles per second; this is not a state reached during hypnosis, which is associated with the alpha and theta states.

Stage One

This is associated with lethargy and the start of relaxation. It is at this point that, to use the old hypnotic cliché, you "are feeling sleepy." In fact, hypnosis is not sleep but this is the time when the hypnotist can induce the first catalepsy. This means some of your muscles begin to feel heavy and you cannot move them. The first area affected is normally the eyelids, where the muscles are small. The hypnotized person's eyes will be shut tight and the subject will feel that he or she doesn't have the strength or energy to open them..

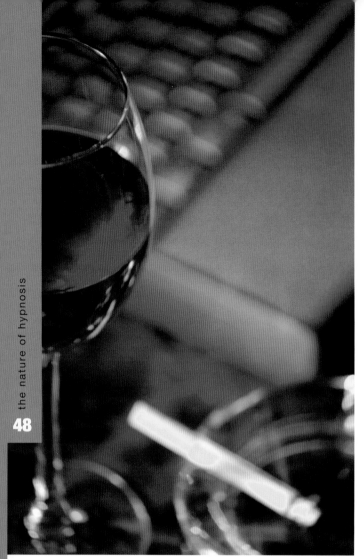

Stage Two

At this level patients will experience catalepsy in particular groups of muscles, for example an arm. They may also have the sensation of being heavy, or of floating. As with Stage One, this level is considered to be a light trance. As the level deepens toward Stage Three, which is considered a medium trance, then the patient may experience catalepsy in both legs or perhaps the whole body.

Stage Three

In the first level of medium trance, as well as experiencing catalepsy the patient can be induced to smell and taste differently. This is where the hypnotist could hold a scented rose underneath the patient's nose and suggest to the subconscious that it smells like an old sock, to which the body will react accordingly. At this level the patient can also be made to discount the existence of a number. For example the hypnotist may suggest that the number three does not exist. When counting to five, the patient would jump straight from two to four, missing three.

Stage Four

Further into a medium trance, the hypnotist can induce amnesia—loss of memory—in the patient. This can be used with post-hypnotic suggestions (regarding the desired changes in the habits or behavior of the patient) to ensure that the patient's conscious mind does not get in the way of the work of the unconscious. Other phenomena include anesthesia—numbness—of parts of the body and analgesia—the state of painlessness.

↪The fourth stage of hypnosis can produce phenomena such as amnesia or loss of memory. At this stage the hypnotist can make post-hypnotic suggestions, which might be used to help give up bad habits such as smoking, drinking, or biting our nails.

Stage Five

This first level of a deep trance is often associated with positive hallucination. This means that the hypnotist can induce the patient to see or hear something that is not there. For example, the hypnotist might say that an empty vase contains a certain type of flower, and the patient will be able to describe it. This is also the level at which stage hypnotists often employ unusual post-hypnotic suggestions so that, when the subject "wakes," he or she might quack like a duck or flap his or her "wings" like a bird.

Stage Six

As this deepest level of trance, patients can experience anesthesia, when surgical operations can be carried out on them. Another phenomenon is negative hallucination, when the patient can be induced not to see or hear things that are really there. Somnambulism—sleepwalking—can also occur at this stage.

These stages are approximate guides to the phenomena experienced under hypnosis, though patients may experience some of them at different times. Also individuals can vary greatly as to how deeply they go into trance and what behavior they display.

Much of the healing work of the hypnotherapist can be carried out in the first three, lighter levels of a trance, which are known as the mnesic (memory-retaining) stages. The second three stages of a deeper trance are often called the amnesic stages.

Hallucination

Hallucination refers to an experience of the physical senses that happens when there is no outside stimulation; in common terms we are "seeing things." In some contexts the term hallucination has bad associations—perhaps with drug-taking or psychotic states. However, hallucinations are also a natural and harmless part of a hypnotic trance. The key distinction is between positive hallucinations and negative hallucinations. In positive hallucinations, the patient in a trance experiences phenomena that are not really present at the time. In negative hallucinations the reverse is true; we are not aware of something that is really there. This latter phenomenon is usually associated with the deepest stages of trance.

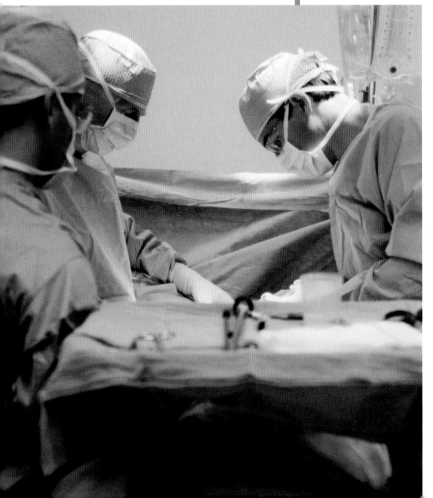

⌣At the deepest forms of trance patients can undergo anesthesia when they not only feel no pain, but are unaware of any physical sensations at all. This stage of trance has been used successfully to carry out surgery on patients.

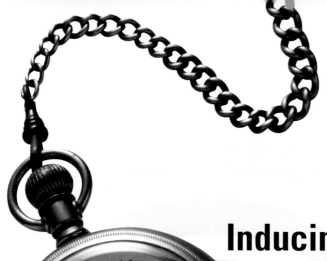

Inducing a trance

If the trance is the key to hypnosis, then the ability to be able to put someone into that trance is obviously very important. This process is usually known as induction. When we go into a trancelike state on our own—for example a daydream—the unconscious is focused on the object of that daydream. However, when someone guides another person into a trance, his or her unconscious is focused on or in communication with the hypnotist. This relationship between the hypnotist and the subject's unconscious is known as rapport. The establishment of a deep rapport between the two is usually regarded as important to success in hypnotherapy. Much of the purpose of the prehypnosis interview between the hypnotist and the subject is to help build up the knowledge and trust of the patient, which will help this rapport develop. The hypnotist will learn the best approach and the best form of words to use for inducing a trance for that particular subject.

↶Ask most people how they think hypnosis is done, and the chances are they will describe a man in a white coat slowly swinging a watch on a chain in front of a patient's eyes. While this was once a common method of inducing a trance, hypnotists now often rely just on words.

There are various techniques used for inducing a trance. The familiar one, and one still strong in the popular concept of hypnosis, is of a man in a white coat swinging a watch slowly in front of the patient's eyes and intoning, "You are feeling sleepy." This technique does work, as it gets the patient concentrating on the movement of the watch. The absorption of the patient's conscious mind by one object is always a key factor in inducing a trance. As the conscious mind is distracted, then the unconscious mind comes to the fore. Another traditional technique is to ask the patient to concentrate on a fixed point on a wall above the eyeline.

Most modern hypnotists use a variety of techniques that build on the more traditional approaches. The older approach of telling subjects they are going into a trance is regarded by some practitioners as being too authoritarian, direct, and rigid to work on some individuals. This is especially true of people who are skeptical about whether they can be put into a trance or not.

The doyen of modern hypnosis, Milton Erickson, developed a new approach to induction in the mid-twentieth century. He came up with more indirect methods, what are called permissive techniques. Though he started off in the 1920s using the direct methods prevalent at the time, Erickson came to understand that a more subtle, less obvious approach worked just as well and often better. The permissive technique involves the hypnotist in using conversation and responding to the subject's reactions. Instead of being told to go into a trance, the subject is gently guided into one.

It is often said by hypnotists that all hypnosis is really self-hypnosis. This means that the hypnotist's main role is to help subjects go into their own hypnotic trance, rather than to hypnotize them. It is we who go into the trance; the hypnotist simply helps us along the way. This is how the permissive technique works, by permitting or allowing the subject to move into a trance.

Ordinary Conversation

One of Erickson's techniques was to engage his client in ordinary conversation before he gradually started using language designed to guide the subject into a trance. The hypnotist might say something like, "Can you experience being more relaxed now?" or "You may have already noticed a change in your breathing," or "As you notice

Inducing a Trance

The methods of helping the subject into hypnosis have varied down through the centuries. The aristocratic Frenchman the Marquis de Puységur—one of the first true hypnotists—seems to have induced a trance by passing his hands over a person's body, as Mesmer had done. The Scotsman James Braid, who invented the term "hypnosis," got his patients to stare at an object such as the case in which he kept his lancet. The nineteenth-century surgeon James Esdaile, who successfully operated on many patients using hypnosis, apparently took hours or sometimes even days before he could get a person into a deep trance ready for surgery. A popular method in the nineteenth century—and one caricatured in the fictional depiction of Svengali—was to use the hypnotist's staring eyes as a means of inducing a trance. Another well-known technique was the use of a watch—swinging or still—to focus subjects' attention.

The general approach was authoritarian, with the hypnotist telling the patient to go into a trance. In the twentieth century, the American Milton Erickson helped pioneer more permissive techniques in which the subject was engaged in conversation that would, often quickly, lead to a trance.

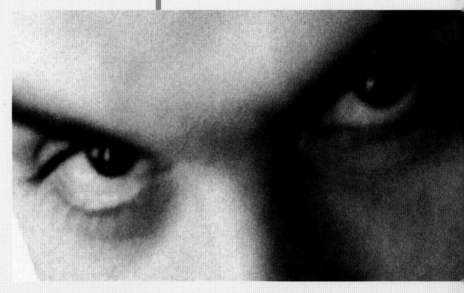

⤳Another false stereotype of hypnosis in the public imagination is that the hypnotist stares into a person's eyes to put him or her into a trance. This was how the fictional character Svengali was said to have performed hypnosis.

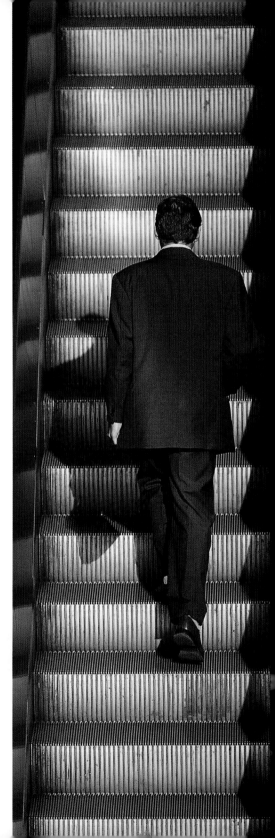

you're now more relaxed, is it easier for you to go into a trance?" What this does is to focus patients' minds on whether they are now more relaxed or breathing differently. The process of doing this helps encourage them into the trance. In this last example there are words and phrases such as "go into a trance," which are embedded into the conversation, and which speak directly to the unconscious mind. The conscious mind may not be aware of it, but the unconscious hears the suggestion.

Erickson believed in responding to everything that happened in the trance, expected or otherwise, and using it to help guide the subject deeper into hypnosis. For example, a patient once asked if Erickson minded if he walked up and down the room during the session. Erickson said he did not, as long as the client allowed him to tell him in which direction to walk. This curious scene went on for around 20 minutes before Erickson directed the man to sit on the chair and go into trance, which he duly did. This technique of adapting surrounding events to the induction is called utilization.

There are many specific induction methods, and individual hypnotists or hypnotherapists tend to develop their own styles. A common one is where the subject is asked to imagine he is slowly walking down stairs, one by one. As the subject's mind sees himself progressing down, he is moving gradually into a deeper and deeper trance.

Another often used method is progressive relaxation. Here, subjects are asked to focus on their heads and gradually feel their muscles relaxing, one by one, progressively down their bodies.

A third common method is for subjects to be asked to count silently backward from, say, 100, concentrating on each number as they say it to themselves.

⤵One method of inducing a trance is to count backward from 100. Other methods rely on repetition and a mental image of a journey (or both). A common one is where the hypnotist asks patients to imagine they are walking slowly down (or up) some stairs. As they move further down (or up) patients are asked to imagine they are going deeper and deeper into a trance.

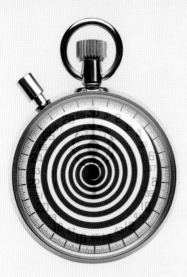

The object of these and other similar techniques is to engage the attention of the conscious mind. By keeping it distracted and preventing it from wandering around with lots of different thoughts, the hypnotist is able to communicate more directly with the unconscious mind.

A more unusual method is the confusion induction. The aim here is to confuse and bewilder the conscious mind and stop it from getting in the way of the trance. This may be achieved by the hypnotist speaking quickly in nonsense language. Soon the conscious mind becomes thoroughly confused by what is going on and gives up trying to understand. As it does, the subject is allowed to move into the hypnotic trance. Though not that common, this approach is sometimes used for skeptical, very logical people whose conscious minds find it hard to switch off during other induction techniques.

The time it takes for a person to "go under" with various induction methods varies between less than a minute to half an hour or more. The length depends on factors such as how relaxed the subject is, how skilled the hypnotist is, how in tune with the client the hypnotist is, and whether the client has been hypnotized before. Someone who is used to the process will generally be induced into a trance more easily.

Once the subject is entering into a trance, the hypnotist will then use similar techniques to deepen the trance, while watching for responses that show just how deep the trance is.

Good therapists will adapt their induction methods to the patient, depending on that person's age and character. They will use their time talking with the client to work out which technique will be most appropriate.

Confusion Induction

One of the ways a hypnotist can bring about a trance in a patient is through a technique sometimes called "confusion induction." It was developed by the great American pioneer of hypnosis, Milton Erickson. The essence of the technique is that the hypnotist is trying to confuse the patient's conscious mind in an attempt to speak directly to the unconscious mind. The hypnotist may create the confusion by starting to talk normally to the patient, then gradually beginning to throw in meaningless words or phrases. He or she may also deliberately use words that don't make sense in the context, use poor grammar or stop sentences half way through, and move onto another subject. When this happens the conscious mind, which is trying to make sense of the world in its rational way, will become confused and distracted. As the patient's conscious mind becomes more intent on trying to make sense of this verbal muddle, it will lose its focus on the outside world, the hypnotist, and the whole idea of being "hypnotized." This is when the hypnotist's words can start to talk directly to the patient's unconscious mind— which responds less to good grammar and complete sentences, but rather to imagination and moods evoked by key words or phrases.

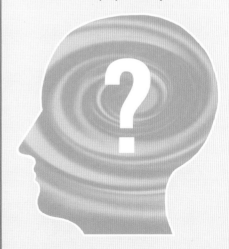

Post-hypnotic suggestions are often used to help cure a patient's bad habits. During a trance the hypnotist suggests to the patient's unconscious mind that—after he or she awakes—whenever he or she has a certain craving or faces a certain situation, he or she will respond in a particular, different way. For example, the suggestion might be that when a person feels stressed or down, instead of having a cigarette he or she takes the dog for a walk.

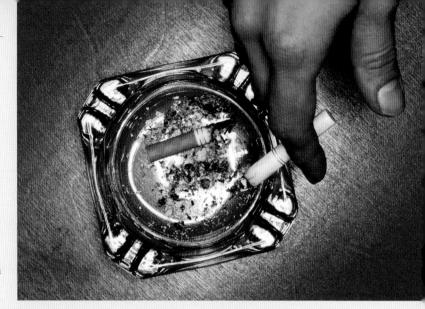

Post-hypnotic suggestions

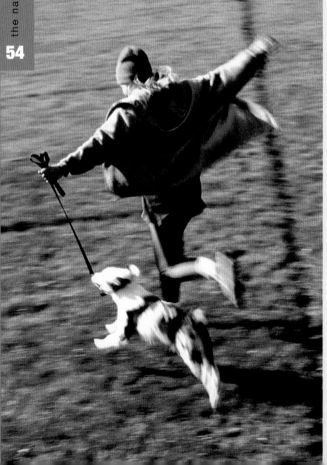

The hypnotic trance is a neutral state. A person who enters a trance and then comes out again may feel more relaxed than usual. But, if the purpose of the trance is to resolve some problem or change a habit, then nothing will alter in the subject unless the unconscious is prompted to change. This is the role of the post-hypnotic suggestion. Hypnotherapists and clinical hypnotists use the patient's trance state to suggest desired changes to the unconscious. They are in effect reprogramming the subconscious mind to change habits and behaviors.

The suggestion is made during the trance with the aim of effecting change that occurs when the patient is out of the trance. Often this is done in the form of suggesting alternative behavior. For example, if someone is trying to give up smoking, the hypnotist may suggest to the patient that when he feels the urge to have a cigarette he will instead eat an apple, drink some water, or have a cup of tea. Or, if the aim of the therapy is to stop eating junk food, then the suggestion might be that, when the subject feels the cravings for this food, she will take the dog for a walk, go for a jog, or do some work in the garden.

The key element of these suggestions is that a negative trait is replaced with a positive one. It is important that something be put in place of the action the patient wants to change. The unconscious mind reacts much better to being told, for example, that a desire to smoke should be replaced by, say, drinking water than to being told simply to stop smoking.

A hypnotist who wants the patient's conscious mind to forget about these trigger suggestions when he awakes will implant them during the amnesic medium or deep trances. When the patient awakes he will be unaware of what the trigger or the suggestion is, but will react to it nonetheless. The reason that hypnotists want the conscious mind to be unaware of the suggestion is so that it will not interfere with it and possibly lessen its effect with doubts.

However, post-hypnotic suggestions can work even if the conscious mind is aware of them. The suggestions that the hypnotist makes can be direct or indirect, command or choice. The "choice," however, may not be real but may be a forced choice between two options, both of which are beneficial. The aim here is to give the subconscious the illusion that it has a choice, when in fact either option may be the desired outcome.

Some hypnotists believe, however, that when a patient is in a deep trance the suggestions should be direct and as clear as possible. Suggestions don't have to be permanent, as they usually are in therapeutic situations; they can be one shot. This is most commonly seen in either research demonstrations or stage hypnosis, when the subject is being instructed to perform a certain act or behave in a specific way.

Suggestion on the Stage

A familiar use of post-hypnotic suggestions is by stage hypnotists. Typically one might see an audience member hypnotized on stage, given a post-hypnotic suggestion, and then returned to his or her seat. Then, at the suggested signal—perhaps the hypnotist scratches his or her left ear or says a certain word—that member of the audience will respond and carry out the activity. This might be to kiss the person sitting next to him or her, or to sing a song. It is important that the hypnotist ensures that the suggestion is removed by the time everyone goes home for the night. Post-hypnotic suggestions last for a variable length of time, and they can wear off. Some researchers have used specific time suggestions, for example that after, say, 18,500 minutes the person will perform a certain action. The results indicate that often the hypnotized person will be remarkably accurate in carrying out the action at the set time. Post-hypnotic suggestion is an aspect of hypnosis that often worries people, who imagine that they might be programmed to behave in an uncharacteristic way. This concern is countered by the argument that no one can be induced to do anything against his or her true wishes, and that this applies equally to post-hypnotic suggestions.

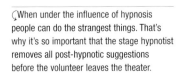

When under the influence of hypnosis people can do the strangest things. That's why it's so important that the stage hypnotist removes all post-hypnotic suggestions before the volunteer leaves the theater.

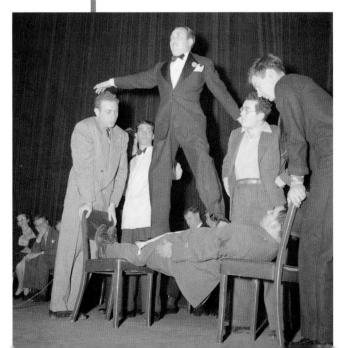

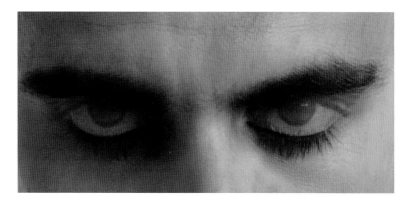

↪A common technique is for the hypnotist to count down slowly from ten. As he or she counts down, the patient will feel as if he or she is coming out of the trance into waking consciousness. The aim is to make the transition as smooth as possible.

♪The traditional method of clicking fingers to signal the end of a trance is still used for dramatic effect by some stage hypnotists. However, many hypnotherapists nowadays consider this to be too sudden.

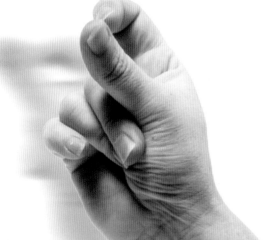

Leaving the Trance

Once the healing suggestions have been made and the purpose of the trance has been accomplished, the final task of the hypnotist is to bring the subject out of that hypnotic state and back into ordinary consciousness.

A traditional method of doing this is for the hypnotist to tell the patient that she will click her fingers at a certain point and that this will bring him out of the trance into a waking state. This is a showmanlike technique still used by some stage hypnotists, because it looks more dramatic. However, many hypnotherapists nowadays consider this method to be too sudden. We have all experienced how being abruptly brought out of a daydream or sleep can be disconcerting. A more common technique is for the hypnotist to tell the patient that she is going to count down slowly from ten. As she counts down, the patient will feel himself slowly coming out of the trance. At the end of the count the patient will be in waking consciousness. Some hypnotists make this process even more gentle by telling patients that they can come to a waking state "in their own time." The aim is to make the transition as smooth as possible. Sometimes, if there is music playing in the background, the patient is instructed to wake from the trance when the music stops.

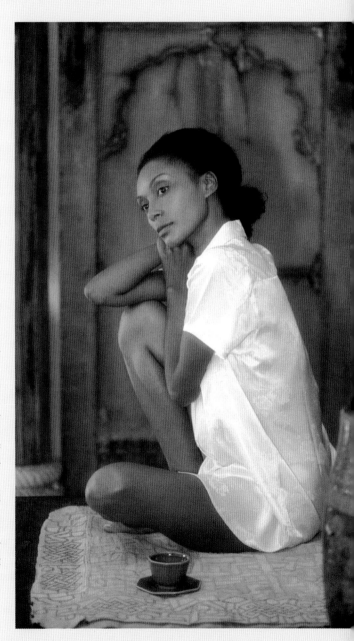

⌒Though hypnosis is not the same as sleep, many people report feeling refreshed and enjoying a general sense of well-being after coming out of a hypnotic trance. Others claim that they sleep better after a session of hypnosis.

The person will remember the hypnosis session afterward, unless a suggestion has been made during the trance to forget it. Often subjects will have a general sense of being relaxed after a session and perhaps a feeling of well-being, but there may well be no other specific signs that tell them they've "been under." Sometimes subjects feel they have been "out" for hours rather than minutes. This is because hypnosis can affect our experience of time. Others may feel refreshed, as if they had just awakened from a long deep sleep, and many report that they sleep much better after a session. It is also quite common for some people to believe that they were never in a trance at all, even though the hypnotist will assure them that they were. On some occasions a patient may have enjoyed the experience so much that he or she may ask when they can have another go. People react in different ways, but hypnotists point out that this is an entirely natural process with no side effects. It is, however, advisable for patients to spend a few minutes gently relaxing before they leave the session for the hurly-burly of the outside world, much as they might after waking from a deep sleep.

During the trance itself the patient will look very relaxed. Sometimes a person's mouth will fall open because the jaw muscles are so relaxed. Very occasionally a patient may drool a little or even shed a few tears, not through sadness but because the tear ducts are relaxed.

Common misconceptions

People are understandably fearful of the unknown. This explains why some are nervous about what a hypnotic trance may involve. A general point that hypnotists make to reassure patients is that a trance is a natural state that we pass through every day, when going into and out of sleep for example. There are also some more specific fears that people have about hypnosis.

Can it be done against my will?

Hypnosis can be a very powerful tool to change your habits, for example to help you give up smoking. But it is not a "magic cure" and is generally only effective if, deep down, you really want to give up smoking or whatever habit it is you want to change. If you do want to change for the better, then hypnosis may well be for you.

The generally accepted view among experts and practitioners is that no person can be hypnotized against his or her wishes.

What about during the trance?

Most hypnotists agree that people cannot be made to do or say anything against their own core beliefs and morals. They point to the fact that to achieve a change in your unconscious behavior you need to want to achieve it. For example, if you do not really want to give up smoking, then a few sessions of hypnosis are unlikely to change your behavior. The subconscious reflects your core beliefs.

Even when stage hypnotists put members of an audience under deep hypnosis and get them to perform unlikely acts such as quacking like a duck, it is argued that the subjects

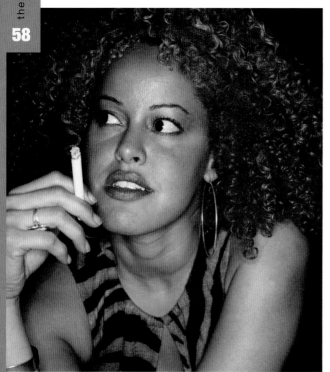

have subconsciously agreed to open themselves up to this; that is, after all, why they agreed to go up on stage.

However, it must be said that, privately, some hypnotists accept that this issue is more complex than it might at first appear. They argue that, by reframing suggestions to make it appear as if they fit in with someone's will, they could make a person do something he or she would not normally do.

The answer to this theoretical risk is that if you do want to visit a hypnotist, then make sure he or she is properly accredited and has a proven track record, and that you take time to speak to and feel you can trust the therapist. Abuses of hypnosis are very rare.

Is hypnosis un-Christian?

There are some Christians who believe that hypnosis is an occult practice and therefore to be avoided. Practitioners point out that hypnosis is a naturally occurring state used as part of therapy to help people. It is therefore neither un-Christian nor pro-Christian, simply a natural medical technique that appears to work. Many Christians both perform hypnosis and have treatment using hypnosis without reporting any concerns. The same applies to other faiths. A person's deep-seated religious faith cannot be affected by hypnosis, unless of course he or she wants it to be.

Will I get stuck?

No. After hundreds of years of the practice, there have been no reports of this. Under hypnosis a person is fully aware, and, if the building where you are sitting starts to burn down or an earthquake occurs, you will quickly come out of the trance. Ultimately, your mind is in control. Some mystics spend many years learning how to stay in a trancelike state, which indicates how difficult that is.

Am I too strong-willed?

A belief that hypnosis is real, and works, does help a person go into a trance and go even deeper. However, a skilled practitioner can overcome the rational doubts of the conscious mind and put someone into a trance, as long as that is what the person wants to happen.

Am I too intelligent?

The evidence suggests that intelligent people are every bit as susceptible to hypnosis as anyone else. Some hypnotists believe that high intelligence can in fact make a person easier to put into a trance.

Will it work for me?

Milton Erickson believed that anyone could be hypnotized. Whether it can help change your habits or behavior will depend on a number of factors, including the skill of your hypnotist, the rapport you have with him or her, your belief that it will work, your desire to change, and the power of your imagination. In other words, it will work if you want it to.

⌡There are a number of modern celebrities who have used hypnosis. One is Kevin Costner who flew out a hypnotist to help him overcome seasickness during the filming of his epic movie, *Waterworld*.

Fear of Hypnosis

It is common for people to fear hypnosis, usually because they know little about it or have been influenced by misleading portrayals in the media. Sometimes trances and hypnosis are said to be associated with magic and the occult. Sometimes they are linked with attempts by organizations and groups to exert mind control techniques over helpless individuals. These associations have little or no foundation in reality. Although organizations such as the CIA did reportedly try to use hypnosis as part of mind control and interrogation experiments after the Second World War, they were soon abandoned. The reason was simple—they didn't work. It is remarkably difficult to get someone to do what they do not, deep down, want to do. The shame is that ingrained fears of hypnosis may deter people from using a very effective therapy. Qualified clinical hypnotists and hypnotherapists help thousands of people each year to overcome phobias of, for example, spiders and heights, gain self-confidence, or quit smoking. If hypnosis was held in less suspicion by the media and the public, even more people might get helped each year.

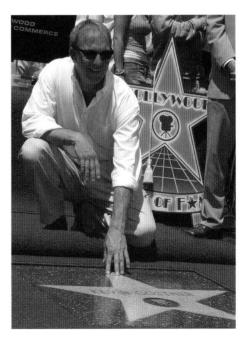

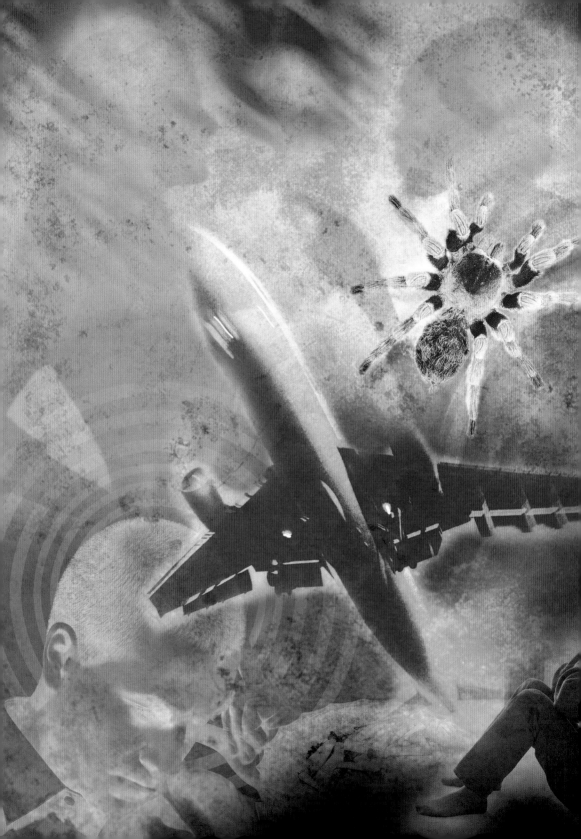

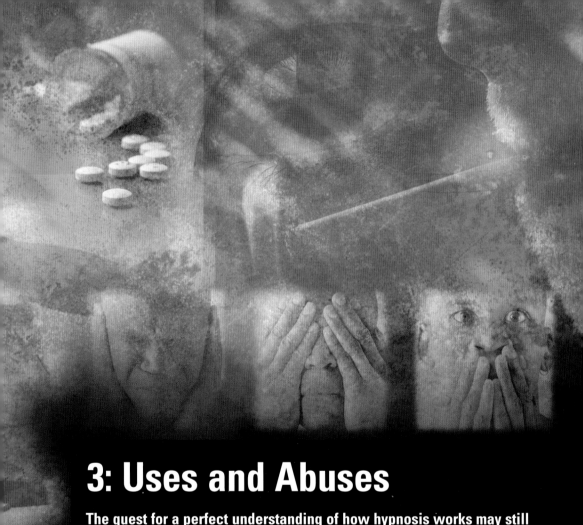

3: Uses and Abuses

The quest for a perfect understanding of how hypnosis works may still go on—but few now doubt that it really works. Whether in helping people to quit smoking, in reducing stress, in improving people's careers, or even in solving crimes, hypnosis has many uses and can have a powerful and beneficial impact on our lives. The use of the technique by so many famous people—from Mozart to Henry Ford—is a telling testament to its power. In wrong or misguided hands, of course, hypnosis can be abused—and this has happened not only among cults and in the scandal of false-memory syndrome, but also in its use by the CIA for hatching plans to create hypnotized assassins

Addictions

Smoking

One of the most common therapeutic uses of hypnosis is to help people stop smoking. There are endless CDs, tapes, and therapy sessions on the market offering hypnosis to help people quit. For many it is the ultimate test of whether hypnosis really works—can it stop someone smoking? The answer seems to be yes. In scientific studies, the use of hypnosis has been shown to be three times as effective as other methods of stopping smoking, with a success rate of about 30 percent. These studies included the use of prerecorded tapes. In one-on-one personal therapy, some hypnotists claim a much higher rate—as much as 95 percent—even with just one session of 90 minutes or less.

The key to the success of hypnosis is that it does not just deal with the addiction to nicotine that afflicts smokers, as other treatments such as patches do. Hypnosis reprograms the unconscious mind to stop the habit of smoking. It can break the link between the trigger activities that smokers associate with having a cigarette.

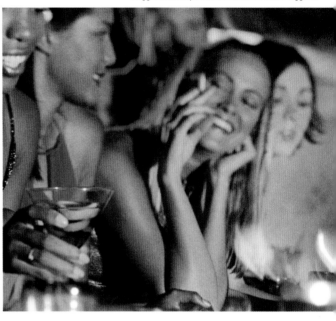

⟲There are many different triggers that can make us want to smoke; it might be visiting a bar with friends for a drink, feeling under stress, or having a ten-minute coffee break. The use of post-hypnotic suggestions helps us react better to those triggers.

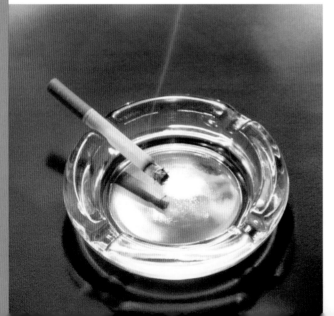

These triggers may include having a cup of coffee, a stressful telephone call, a business meeting, or having just eaten a meal; each smoker may have one or more such triggers that prompt him or her to smoke. The associations between these triggers and the habit of smoking exist in the unconscious mind, and remain even after the physical addiction to nicotine has gone. However, when the hypnotist makes the right suggestions to the smoker's unconscious, these powerful associations are removed or, better still, replaced.

The hypnotist will find out what an individual's own triggers are and associate them with healthier habits. The therapist will suggest to the unconscious that, when the patient feels the urge to smoke, she will drink water, eat some fruit, do some exercises, or phone a sympathetic ex-smoker for support. Often the suggestions will focus on the benefits of not smoking—better health, improved sense of taste, more money—rather than on the negative effects of continuing the habit. After treatment the patient will usually be advised to avoid the triggers to smoking for a few days, including meetings with smokers in social situations where she might be tempted to have "just one" cigarette with a friend. After a short period, however, the patient is usually able to resume normal behavior as the association between the smoking triggers and smoking is broken. This includes spending time with people who still smoke. Hypnotists commonly implant a suggestion that the patients will be tolerant of other people's smoking, but will not themselves feel the urge to smoke.

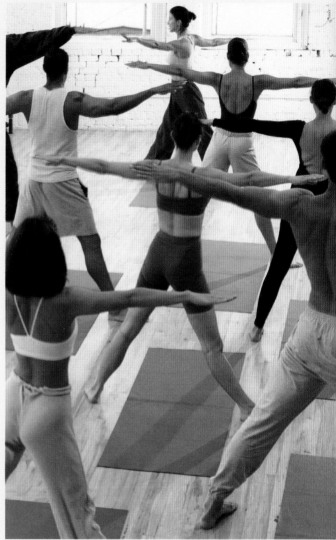

Hypnosis aimed at curing bad habits is far more effective if it seeks to replace the bad habit with a good one. For example, the hypnotist will implant the suggestion that the patient will want to take some exercise, eat fruit, or drink water—rather than having a smoke, eating too much sweet food, or whatever his or her bad habit is.

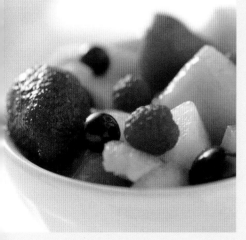

Alcoholism

The use of hypnosis to treat alcohol addiction is much less widespread than with smoking, though some practitioners do offer this treatment. This may in part be because the underlying causes of alcoholism are more complex and varied than those of smoking. These causes may include depression, low self-esteem, and insecurity in social situations. Hypnosis is able to tackle some of these problems, for example by making a patient feel more confident in social gatherings to remove the urge to drink alcohol to feel "braver." And there have been some cases in which hypnosis has successfully stopped an alcoholic from drinking, using suggestions over a number of sessions to build up self-esteem, and informing the unconscious mind that the subject no longer enjoys alcohol. However, hypnosis is rarely used as a stand-alone treatment for alcoholism. More commonly, hypnosis is used together with other forms of treatment, provided through Alcoholics Anonymous (AA) meetings, for example, or by a medical practitioner. In such cases hypnosis can be used to strengthen a person's determination to undergo treatment, or to continue with it once he or she has started. Hypnosis used in this way can be a very powerful tool in helping to overcome alcohol addiction.

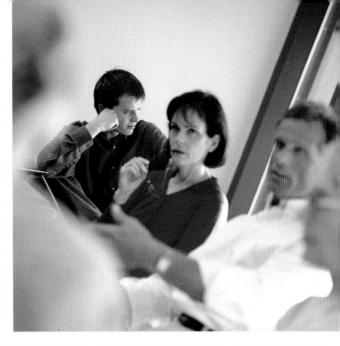

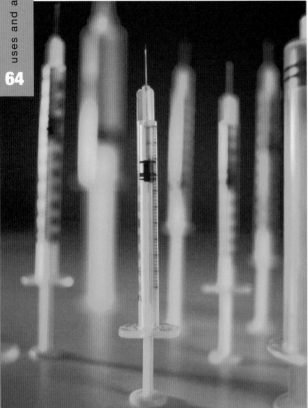

Hypnosis can be a valuable tool in helping to overcome alcohol or drug addiction, but it is rarely used as the sole therapy in such cases. More often hypnosis will be used to help strengthen the patient's resolve to get and maintain specialist help, whether through Alcoholics Anonymous or in drug rehabilitation programs.

Drugs

Hypnosis is sometimes employed to help drug addicts gain the mental resolve to undergo proper treatment for their addiction. Very often, addicts may feel they want to stop, but at the same time fear they do not have the strength to go through with the treatment. This is where hypnosis can help. During a trance, a hypnotist will suggest to the addict's unconscious that the subject wants to have treatment, is looking for change, and has a desire to get better.

However, simply implanting the suggestion that a person give up drugs can be dangerous, for example if a physical dependence on the substance has developed. Hypnosis may help with the psychological dependence on a drug, but not necessarily with the physical addiction. As a result, and as with alcoholics, hypnosis for drug addicts is nearly always performed in conjunction with treatment by a medical practitioner.

Overeating

Next to smoking, eating too much is one of the most widespread harmful habits in modern western society. It can lead to obesity, and a variety of health and social problems. The unfair part is that, while some people can seemingly eat as much as they want without putting on so much as an ounce in weight, others can pile on the pounds very easily. For these individuals the constant cycle of diets, watching the pounds go back on, then yet more dieting, can be grim. It is hard to change these eating habits, and the sad fact is that many people who succeed in losing weight through a diet eventually do put that weight back on again.

Hypnosis can help people trapped in this vicious cycle by reprogramming their unconscious minds to want less food, to eat less fattening foods, and to think and behave like a thin person. Powerful suggestions can be implanted during a trance to stop the patient from wanting to snack between meals, or eat junk food, or eat candy while watching television or surfing the Internet. Instead, these habits will be replaced with new ones, such as eating fruit, drinking water, taking exercise, or taking the dog for a walk. Used together with a diet program, hypnosis can be a very effective tool for permanent weight loss.

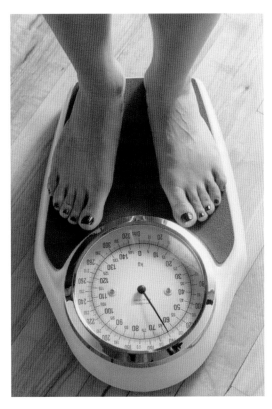

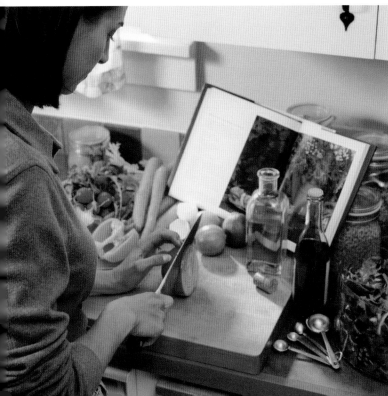

⌒For people with a weight problem, hypnosis can be employed to help them start to "think thin." Used together with a sensible diet, hypnosis can be of real benefit for someone trying to lose all those unwanted pounds.

Phobias

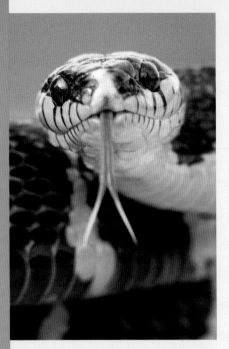

Phobias can make our lives a misery. To the outsider these fears appear—and indeed are—utterly illogical and irrational. To the person with the phobia, however, the fear is all too real. There are many, many different phobias; in fact, a person can have a phobia about almost anything. Common ones include fear of flying, fear of rodents, fear of heights, fear of insects, fear of open spaces, and fear of confined spaces. Others include a phobia of crossing the road, oceans, computers, cats, dogs, snakes—the list goes on and on. Very often the phobia is obscure enough that we don't have to worry too much about it. For example, if you have a morbid fear of mountains, but spend all your life on the Florida coast, this phobia is unlikely to cause you many problems. Similarly, having an irrational fear of cows is not going to be a big handicap to your life if you live in downtown Manhattan, London, or Sydney. But very often phobias such as fear of flying, fear of elevators, and fear of open spaces, can be major obstacles to living a normal life. In most cases, hypnosis is a very effective tool for removing these irrational fears, and more and more people are turning to the treatment for help.

Phobias can come in all shapes and sizes. Some of them, such as a morbid fear of snakes, may not be too much of a problem, especially if you live in areas where you are unlikely to encounter them. But phobias of, for example, being in open spaces, flying in airplanes, or taking elevators, can be a major obstacle to having a normal life in modern society. Hypnosis can be a remarkably effective treatment.

The Object of the Fear

One technique used by hypnotherapists is to get patients to come to terms, step by step, with the object of their fear. During a trance, clients will be asked to imagine or visualize the object of their fear at a safe distance. For example, someone with a cat phobia might be asked to imagine a cat on the other side of town, far enough away so

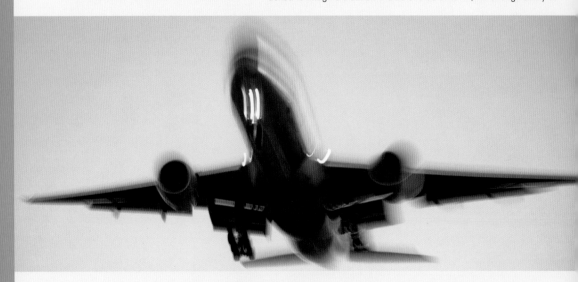

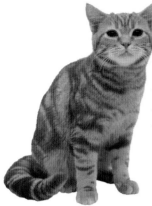

In hypnosis sessions the object of fear, such as a cat, is visualized closer and closer to the patient. Eventually the patient visualizes himself or herself stroking it—without fear.

she can visualize it without distress. Gradually, and over a few sessions, the patient would visualize the cat closer and closer to her, without it causing her any distress. Hypnotic suggestions would reassure her that she had no problem with cats, that the cat was no threat to her, in fact, that she was fond of cats. Eventually, the patient would visualize herself close to the animal, touching it, and feeling no anxiety. The phobia would be defeated.

Another approach is to take the patient back, through regression, to the time when the phobia first developed. Sometimes, though not invariably, a phobia was caused by a trigger event from earlier in our lives, which we may have forgotten. We may have been bitten by a dog or been shut up in a closet by older siblings. During a trance the hypnotist will take the patient back to before this trigger event and make him aware of what it felt like before he had the phobia. The hypnotist will then use this feeling to replace the patient's phobia with a more positive frame of mind. Just being consciously aware of the trigger event can sometimes be enough to remove the phobia.

Hypnotists do have to be careful how they tackle phobias. For example, someone with a phobia about snakes does not want to have all inhibitions about them removed to the extent that she would cheerfully pick up a rattlesnake. This is why therapists take care to listen to patients. A patient will not perhaps want to enjoy the company of poisonous snakes but want simply not to have an unreasonable fear about them.

Similarly, hypnosis can be used to help treat a variety of other disorders, including panic disorders, obsessive-compulsive disorder, and post-traumatic stress disorder.

The Case of the Gerbil Phobia

The hypnosis method for dealing with phobias does not always have to be gradual. In one recent case a young woman went to a hypnotist worried because she had been asked to look after a young relative's pet gerbil during a vacation break. The problem was, the woman had a morbid fear of gerbils and other rodents. Even worse, the vacation began the next day, so there was no time for a lengthy series of sessions. Undeterred, the hypnotist put his patient into a trance and suggested to her unconscious that she actually quite liked gerbils, and moreover she was even looking forward to caring for her relative's pet. Her mind seems to have been successfully reprogrammed—the gerbil-sitting continued for many years to come. This case illustrates how successful hypnosis can be in dealing with phobias.

Fear of Vegetables

One therapist had a 30-year-old client who suffered from lachanophobia—fear of vegetables. Not only could she not eat vegetables, but she was upset because she could not even prepare them for her children. The very smell of vegetables brought on a panic attack. Under hypnosis, she spontaneously recalled that, when she was about six, her mother was giving all her attention to her new baby; she apparently fought her mother on the issue of eating vegetables in order to regain her mother's attention. Part of her felt that if she ate vegetables again without a fuss, she would lose her mother's love. With the use of suggestion, the therapist was able to get her first to buy some carrots, then to eat them. Eventually, the therapy created a normal approach to vegetables.

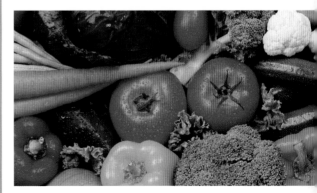

Home truths

Shyness

Many, if not most of us, have experienced shyness at some points in our lives. It may have been while meeting someone we admired or someone to whom we were physically attracted, or when being asked to address a group of complete strangers. Much of the time it is something we have quickly gotten over and forgotten about, and it has not become a major issue in our lives. On occasions, a certain level of shyness can even be an attractive and desirable trait.

There are people, though, for whom deep shyness is a serious problem. For these people, the very idea of speaking to a stranger at a party, asking questions in a class, walking in a crowd, or opening the door to the mailman, may cause anxiety. Even the thought of eating in a public place such as a restaurant may be too much for them. They blush, their palms feel sweaty, and they start to panic. It is often a hidden condition, and individuals might do their best to hide it from friends or even their family. At its worst, such crippling shyness is like a phobia and can ruin a person's life. This level of fear is often associated with low self-esteem and a lack of confidence.

Hypnosis can be of enormous benefit to people who suffer this much-overlooked condition. Though genetics may have a role to play in causing extreme shyness, it is also to an extent a learned behavior; a behavior

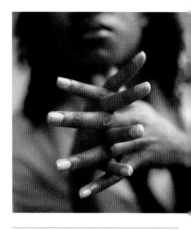

For many people shyness is one of those things that happens every now and again, but does not become a major issue. However, for a few people extreme shyness can be crippling. Hypnotherapy can be a powerful tool for helping a person to overcome this extreme timidity, and to learn how to cope with social situations.

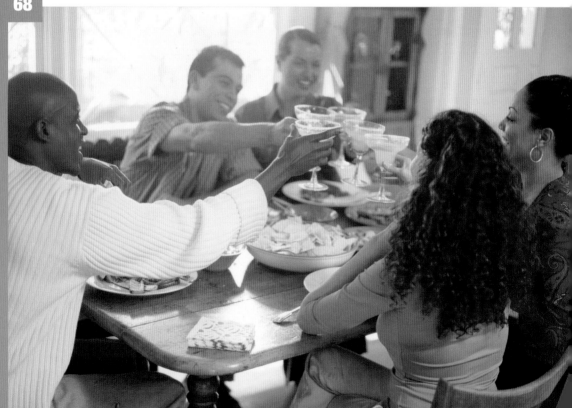

working at the unconscious level. That is the bad news. The good news is that it is possible for the unconscious to learn, or be taught, new behavior.

The therapist's approach may be to get the patient to visualize himself in certain social situations and to see himself feeling and behaving in a more confident manner. The suggestions to the unconscious mind will tell the patient that he has a great deal to offer, that his opinions are important, that he can contribute to the world around him. Gradually the person's self-esteem will increase and will begin to be reflected in his behavior. In turn, each little success gained in overcoming his shyness can be used to boost his confidence even more, creating a "virtuous cycle."

Difficulty with Relationships

Our ability to make friends can be affected by our social timidity. In these cases the hypnotist can work with a patient in much the same way as for shyness. The patient's confidence will be boosted, and she will imagine herself able to meet and make new friends with greater ease.

Another role for hypnosis, however, is in helping *existing* relationships. Often relationships and marriages can go through difficult patches for no obvious reasons. Or perhaps a fierce difference of opinion between two otherwise good friends might create an unseen barrier between them. The same can be true of relationships within families, where long-forgotten and trivial arguments can set relatives apart. Hypnosis is often used to overcome these difficulties. During a trance, the patient's view of the problematic relationship can be reframed so that she sees it in a new light. Both old and new issues can be confronted and overcome by allowing the patient to see that the underlying relationship is strong. This therapy is, of course, much more effective if both parties agree to undergo it.

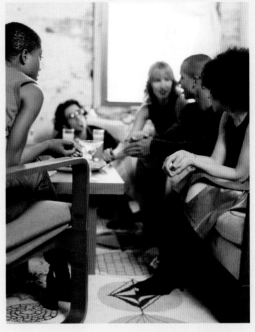

⤵It can be hard for some people to make friends. As for shyness, hypnotherapy can be used to help explore the reasons for this timidity and then to help boost confidence in forming relationships with others.

⤵Close personal relationships, including marriages, can begin to fall apart even without us realizing it or knowing why. A hypnotherapist will enable clients to discover the causes of tensions, and encourage them to resolve these. Sometimes the therapy will uncover grievances that our conscious minds have long forgotten, but which are lodged in our unconscious minds.

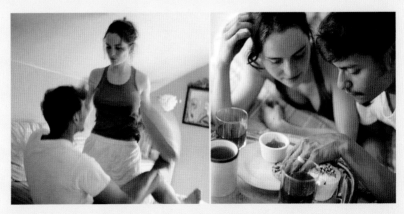

Bad Habits

It is quite common for people to worry. Most of us do worry about something, though usually the worry passes and we think about something else. An occasional worry is natural, often useful, and sometimes necessary. People who never seem to have a care in the world can even seem very irritating to the rest of us. Some people, however, become consumed by worry. We are not talking about fully fledged medical conditions, but about people who simply worry about things too much. Even though they may know consciously

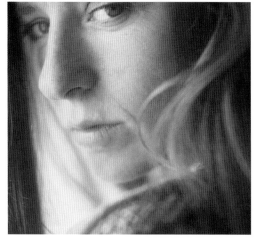

that thinking or worrying about a problem will not change anything, it does not stop them. They become trapped in a world of endless anxiety, always finding something else to concern them, even if an existing problem is suddenly solved. For them, worry has become a habit, a way of looking at the world, and the more they worry, the more it comes to be a deep-seated habit—a vicious circle. The good news is that, like any habit, it can be changed and replaced with a new and better one. The approach of the hypnotist is to tackle any specific worries head on, suggesting to the unconscious mind solutions or explanations. At the same time, the underlying tendency to worry will be explored, and posthypnotic suggestions offered to help the client change to a more positive outlook.

Physical bad habits, such as nail biting and hair pulling, can also be treated with hypnosis. Often a hypnotist will use a simple suggestion to the unconscious that each time the person feels an urge to bite his nails he will do something else—for example, smile or have a happy thought. The unconscious mind seems to react better to suggestions when these replace one habit with another, rather than just removing the bad habit. Nature abhors a vacuum.

⌣Worry and anxiety can be extremely draining. While most of us may suffer this experience for only short periods, for a few of us worry is all-consuming. It becomes a habit, and we may even forget what the original source of our concern was. Hypnosis can unlock those reasons and allow our unconscious mind to overcome the constant anxiety.

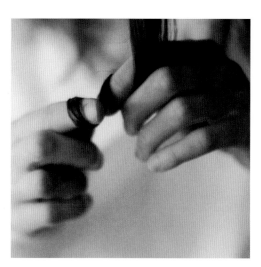

☽Biting our nails or pulling our hair are nervous habits that can irritate us or even others. The use of hypnosis can replace the urge to perform these bad habits with good ones.

Insomnia

Sleep is something we all need. Being unable to get to sleep or waking up habitually early can make us feel tired and stressed throughout the day. Hypnosis is frequently performed as a highly successful treatment for sleep problems. During a trance, the hypnotist suggests to the patient that she will sleep easily and throughout the night, and that she will awaken at the normal time feeling relaxed and refreshed. Sometimes the hypnotist will suggest trigger points that will induce sleep, such as holding the pillow in a certain way or facing in a certain direction. Therapists will be careful, though, to suggest that patients will awake when they have to; they do not want to discourage necessary visits to the bathroom, for example. If an emergency such as a fire occurs, a person will naturally awaken anyway, thanks to the human instinct for self-preservation. The unconscious mind acts in the way it believes best protects and preserves the individual.

Another technique is for clients to visualize themselves asleep in their bed as time passes, seeing how they are getting a good night's sleep, and embedding this suggestion in the unconscious mind.

Nightmares, too, can be resolved by hypnosis. A simple suggestion can tell the unconscious that when the bad dream starts a different ending will occur, that the client will switch to another, nicer dream, or maybe become a hero and alter the outcome.

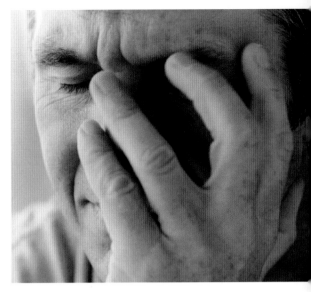

⤸Few things are more debilitating than insomnia. We all need a good night's sleep, and hypnosis can be one of the best therapies for ensuring that we get one.

⤹Using hypnosis, the patient will not only learn how to get to sleep at night, but thanks to the power of suggestion she will often find she wakes up feeling even more rested than usual.

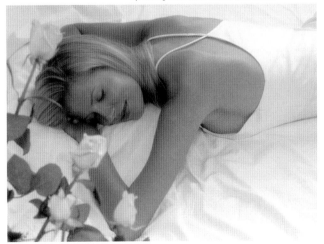

Jackie Kennedy Onassis

Jacqueline Kennedy Onassis (1929–1994) led a remarkable life in which she experienced considerable tragedy. Most tragic of all, of course, was the assassination of her husband, President John F. Kennedy, in Dallas on November 22, 1963, at which Mrs. Kennedy herself was present. Then her second husband, the Greek businessman Aristotle Onassis, died in 1975, just seven years after they were married. Jackie Kennedy Onassis is said to have used hypnotherapy to "relive and let go of" some of these tragic events in her life, and it is thought to have brought her considerable comfort. Sometimes the process of confronting past experiences and fears during a trance is enough to allow a person to come to terms with them.

Work and art

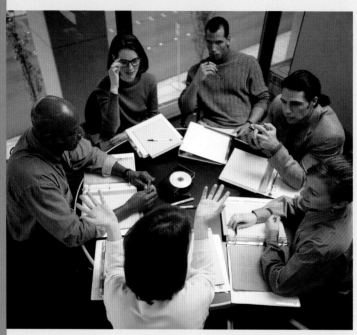

↩Hypnosis is now being used in workplaces and in market research with impressive results. The technique can help people relax and say what they really feel in focus groups; while at work meetings it can ensure that everyone is happy to have his or her say, rather than allowing one or two strong characters to dominate proceedings. This means a company makes full use of its biggest asset—its staff.

Careers

Practical applications of hypnosis are not confined to our personal lives. More and more people are now using the technique to help them in their jobs and careers. The technique is useful for people who want to improve their interview techniques, public-speaking skills, relations with colleagues, or memory skills. Some salespeople use visualizing and self-confidence suggestions during a trance to help them clinch deals. Others use hypnosis to enable them to be more assertive with management, perhaps to ask for a raise or a promotion. On occasion, employees are nervous about being able to keep up with new training regimes or use new equipment. Posthypnotic suggestions are used to allay those fears and reassure them that they will be able to cope with whatever they are asked to do.

Problems in the office environment can arise from interstaff relations, in other words, office politics. It can be easy for workers to get things out of proportion in the pressure-cooker atmosphere of work. Staff may be encouraged to undergo hypnosis to learn strategies for coping with such tensions, which will enable them to concentrate on their jobs.

Giving Everyone a Say

A fascinating new use of hypnosis is with groups of employees in staff brainstorming sessions and in focus groups. In the brainstorming sessions, hypnosis helps remove any inhibitions staff might have in putting forward their ideas, no matter how unusual they might be. This is especially useful for groups where a few strong individuals overshadow others, or in companies where people are afraid to talk up in front of the boss. The hypnotized focus groups also benefit from this greater equality of voice. Moreover, the emphasis on the unconscious mind's reaction removes the inhibitions of our conscious mind and helps the focus group members be more honest about the brands being discussed. Sometimes, age regression is used in these sessions to discover when the members of the group first came across a brand and in what circumstances. This is useful for a company in understanding their product's core appeal and how it engages—or does not engage—with our unconscious mind.

Artists, Writers, and Composers

Throughout history, artists have used hypnosislike trances to inspire their craft. The list includes the composers Mozart and Chopin, as well as the German poet Goethe, and the British poet Tennyson. Nowadays, many writers, artists, and musicians use hypnosis to boost their creativity. The fast pace and pressures of modern life can be a substantial obstacle to the creative process. Hypnosis can help artists get in touch with their creative urges. Of course, hypnotic suggestions put to artists in trances do not magically give them the talent to write, paint, or compose to a level they were not able to before. Instead, they ensure that the existing creativity of the artist is not blocked by doubts or problems. In the case of a writer, for example, hypnosis might be able to cure the phenomenon known as writer's block.

Some hypnotists also claim to be able to use hypnotic suggestion to enable anyone to achieve perfect musical pitch. This is a wonderful idea, though it must be said the evidence for the claim is purely anecdotal.

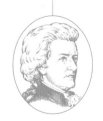

Wolfgang Amadeus Mozart

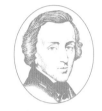

Frédéric François Chopin

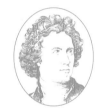

Johann Wolfgang von Goethe

The Arts

The great composer Frédéric François Chopin (1810–1849) had a great interest in hypnosis, so much so that he enrolled for classes in the subject at the University of Strasbourg. Another student was the brilliant German poet, writer, and scientist Johann Wolfgang von Goethe (1749–1832). Other great artists who have used hypnosis include the Russian composer Sergei Rachmaninov (1873–1943), who suffered composer's block after writing his Symphony No. 1 in 1897. In desperation he turned to hypnosis and underwent three months of sessions with the hypnotist Nikolai Dahl. Dahl used suggestions to persuade the Russian composer that he would indeed be able to resume composition. As a result, Rachmaninov wrote his Piano Concerto No. 2, one of his most acclaimed works, and a composition dedicated to his therapist. Another artist who used hypnosis was the great British poet Alfred, Lord Tennyson (1809–1892), who used to repeat words to himself rather like a mantra, to alter his state of consciousness; whole poems would come to him while he was in this state.

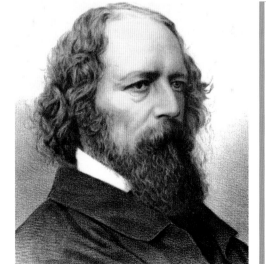

Alfred Lord Tennyson

Ford and Einstein

The father of the modern automobile industry, Henry Ford (1863–1947), was said to have used hypnosis to improve his life. Certainly there is no doubt that one of the most successful and visionary businessmen in history knew the power of the mind. The brilliant physicist and mathematician Albert Einstein (1879–1955), who came up with the special and general theories of relativity, also understood the power of the mind and was said to have used hypnosislike trances for inspiration. He once said, "Imagination is more important than knowledge." Imagination and suggestion are two critical ingredients of successful hypnosis.

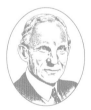

Henry Ford

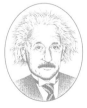

Albert Einstein

Medical matters

The application of clinical hypnosis to treating specific physical diseases and conditions is still in its infancy. Some hypnotists see no reason why, in theory, suggestions made to the unconscious mind should not be able to help treat major illnesses such as cancer and HIV. As yet, however, the evidence that hypnosis can be effective with such major illnesses is anecdotal. But with other medical conditions there is already compelling evidence that hypnosis does have a serious role, not just in alleviating, but also in removing symptoms altogether.

⌒Allergies are a growing feature of modern life. All around there are small particles, such as pollen (pictured), some of which may trigger reactions from our immune systems. Hypnotists claim a high success rate—up to 80 percent—in curing most kinds of allergy.

Irritable Bowel Syndrome

Irritable bowel syndrome (IBS) is one of the most common medical complaints in modern life. It is estimated that more than 4.5 million Americans alone suffer from this discomforting and painful complaint of the digestive system. Though there are a number of different treatments for IBS, hypnosis is emerging as one of the most popular. This form of treatment has a success rate of more than 80 percent, according to recent studies. As with all the other treatments, hypnosis does not cure IBS—there is no cure at present—but it does help alleviate the symptoms. The patients are put into hypnotic trance and encouraged to take control of their bodies through the workings of their unconscious mind.

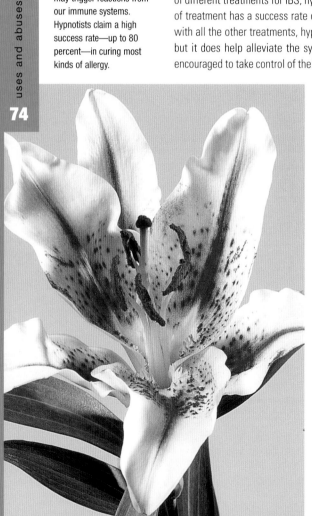

Allergies

Allergies are a major feature of modern life. Just about everyone suffers or knows someone who suffers from a form of allergy, be it to pollen, certain kinds of food, milk, or cats. Indeed, some people are said to be allergic to modern life and the chemicals and substances that surround us all. Hypnosis is increasingly used to treat everyday allergies, and, though the results are as yet largely anecdotal, some hypnotists claim success rates of around 80 percent. The theory is that many allergies are caused when the body's immune system mistakes the pollen, or whatever the allergen is, for a potentially dangerous substance. Hypnosis aims to reprogram the immune system's response to the allergen via the unconscious mind. Gradually, patients are persuaded under a trance that their bodies have nothing to fear from the allergen and should stop the allergic reaction, the production of histamines with which we associate the sneezing, red eyes, and runny noses of allergy.

Cancer

Hypnosis has had a role in cancer treatment for a number of years. However, this use has largely been restricted to helping to give patients the determination to continue with the often stressful medical treatment that cancer therapy entails. There is certainly some strong anecdotal evidence that hypnosis can alleviate some of the hardships of cancer treatment such as chemotherapy, as well as reducing the negative thoughts and doubts that cancer patients frequently feel. It can also help reduce the pain of cancer itself.

Much more controversial are the claims that, through hypnosis, the unconscious mind can be trained to attack the cancer and ultimately help cure patients. This approach fits in with the theory that the unconscious mind governs the body's immune system, the function of the body that leads the fight against cancerous cells. So far, however, there have been no studies that demonstrate this. In any case, any qualified hypnotist contacted by a cancer patient will ensure that the client has sought conventional medical treatment for the illness, and will try to work in harmony with conventional therapy.

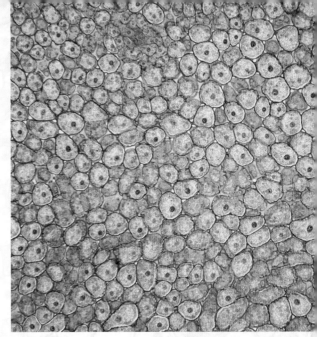

◡In therapy that uses hypnosis the patients are asked to use their imagination—the language of the unconscious mind—to help deliver their goals. In cancer cases, for example, patients are asked to visualize their immune system fighting and killing the cancer cells, shown here.

Other Illnesses

Claims have been made that hypnosis can help in the treatment of other serious medical conditions, including assisting patients who are HIV-positive and those who have high blood pressure or have suffered a stroke. It is highly likely that hypnosis can help with boosting the mental strength of a person to cope with the diagnosis of HIV as well as with alleviating some of the physical symptoms. Anecdotal evidence also suggests that hypnotic suggestions can help patients lower their blood pressure; and some intriguing initial research has shown that hypnosis may help in the recovery of stroke patients. In the latter example, the hypnotist effectively reminds the subconscious of what the body used to be able to do and suggests that it can do it again. In all cases, however, it is important that sufferers seek help from a medical practitioner. Hypnosis may be extremely effective, but it should not be regarded as a miracle wonder cure.

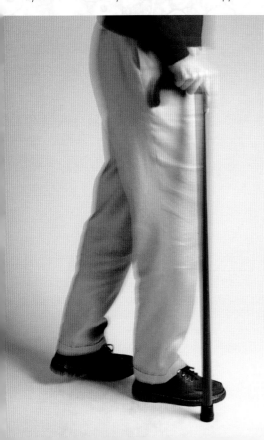

◡Although not a miracle cure, the use of hypnosis in the recovery of stroke patients is being researched.

Pain relief

In 2000, researchers at Beth Israel Deaconess Medical Center in Boston found that hypnosis was able to reduce both surgical pain and surgery time, and improve safety. In a trial of 241 patients, it was discovered that patients who used self-hypnotic relaxation techniques during surgery generally needed less pain medication and left the operating room sooner. They also had more stable vital signs during the operation.

This study backed up what supporters of hypnosis have long maintained—that potentially one of the most important benefits of hypnosis is in the control of pain. Already, a number of hospitals around the world are beginning to use hypnosis to reduce pain and discomfort from surgery and other medical techniques. In the mid-nineteenth century, pioneers such as James Braid and James Esdaile had used hypnosis to carry out major surgery. However, the advent of chemical anesthesia meant that the surgical applications of hypnosis were then left unexplored for decades.

Pain is something we all experience in our lives. When our body undergoes a pain-causing experience, this message is passed through our nervous system to our brain, which then causes us to feel pain. Therefore, pain has a useful purpose in telling us something is wrong. If a child did not feel the onset of pain when he puts his hand close to a flickering flame, he might be tempted to continue—with disastrous results.

No Side Effects

However, anyone who has had to live with constant or recurring pain knows just how debilitating this can be. Of course, one can use painkilling drugs, which are often very effective. But they can be expensive and they do have side effects. The advantage of hypnosis is that it has no side effects. Pain relief through hypnosis has, for example, been used very effectively in some burns units in the United States.

In tackling pain, one technique is for the hypnotist to suggest directly to the patient's unconscious mind that the pain is getting less and ultimately disappearing. This induces what is called analgesia—when the body can experience sensations but does not feel pain. Another approach is where the patient is made to dissociate from the pain. The hypnotist will ask her to imagine the pain as a separate color, shape, or object, and then visualize this object gradually disappearing, perhaps by floating up in a balloon or shrinking in size.

With recurring pain attacks such as migraine headaches, the therapist may use hypnosis to relieve

> Since the eighteenth and nineteenth centuries, hypnotists have grasped the extraordinary power of hypnosis to control pain in patients. This aspect of hypnosis is now being used more and more in modern surgery as a practical alternative to chemical anesthetics.

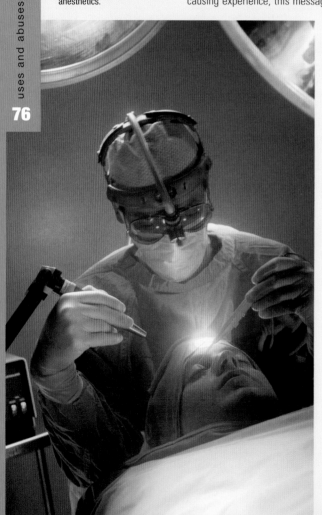

Pain is unpleasant, of course, but it does perform a useful function in our lives. Pain, for example, tells us when our body is being harmed and warns us that we need to take action to avoid more damage. But in surgery or in cases of chronic pain, it is desirable to control the pain as much as possible. The experience of pain is passed through our body and nerves, through the spinal cord, and on to a receptor in the brain. In hypnosis the aim is to persuade the mind that it is not receiving the message of pain, even though the body is still aware of the pain-causing sensation. This phenomenon is known as analgesia.

Brain receives pain message

Signals transmitted along a pathway of the spinal cord

Pain signals sent to spine

Acute pain

Operating under Hypnosis

In 1994 a British man, Andy Bryant, demonstrated the potential usefulness of hypnosis for pain control when he underwent a vasectomy operation without anesthesia. Before the surgery, the 36-year-old hairdresser put himself into a hypnotic trance and said he felt "great" after the brief four-minute operation in Central London.

Andy explained afterward: "You can feel the sensation of the knife cutting, but you switch the pain off." He said he had known what to expect, as he had earlier had an operation on his toes while under hypnosis. Although on this occasion Andy took his own hypnotist along, he ended up hypnotizing himself in ten minutes before the vasectomy took place. In the nineteenth century, one of James Esdaile's patients had a tumor weighing more than 100 pounds removed from his body while under hypnosis—without feeling anything.

the pain, and then teach the patient self-hypnosis so he can deal with the discomfort if and when a migraine attack reoccurs. It should be remembered, however, that, because pain is a sign that something may be wrong, a patient should seek medical advice to deal with the cause of the pain as well as using hypnosis to alleviate it.

In a deep trance, patients can experience anesthesia, in which they feel no sensations at all. In such a state it is possible for a person to undergo major surgery without feeling pain. This is especially useful in dental work, where patients may be unwilling to have injections or nitrous oxide when undergoing major operations. The advantage again is that there are no side effects (such as a numb mouth) or any risk from general anesthetic.

Hypnosis is used to overcome a person's fear of going to the dentist in the first place, a fairly common phobia among many adults. It can also be employed as a way of reducing a patient's bleeding during a dental procedure such as the removal of a tooth. Reports indicate that, if it is suggested to the unconscious mind that the patient will bleed less during an operation, then this is precisely what happens.

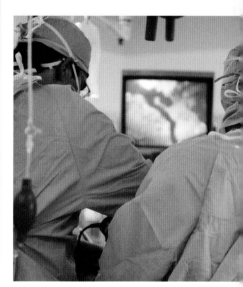

Childbirth and pregnancy

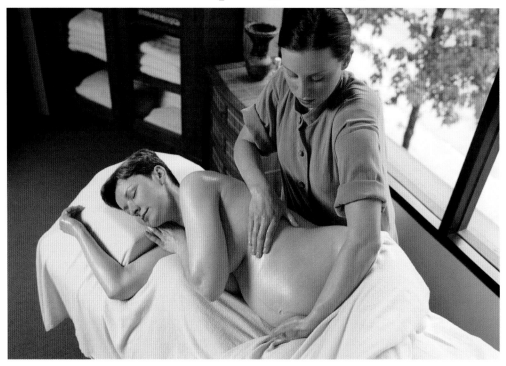

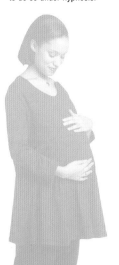

◗One of the most painful experiences in a woman's life can be childbirth, which is why so many women understandably look for the most pain-free ways of giving birth. One of these is to do so under hypnosis.

Giving birth to a child is one of the most natural events in the world, but it can also be one of the most painful. Women want to experience the wonder of childbirth—but are understandably concerned at having to deal with its painful effects. This explains why expectant mothers are always on the hunt for the most natural way of giving birth that also alleviates the discomfort. This search for new techniques explains the current interest in giving birth under hypnosis.

According to one study at the University of Wisconsin in Canada, women who had received instruction in hypnosis for childbirth experienced shorter labors and reduced pain. This was compared with a control group that had taken part in regular prenatal classes in which they learned standard breathing and relaxation techniques. The benefits of hypnosis during childbirth are not just reduced pain and shorter labors. It can also mean less medication is required, which in turn means the mental recovery time after births can be much quicker as well. One of the greatest attractions of using the technique is that the woman remains mentally alert during the delivery, and can be fully aware of this life-changing experience.

Experts who teach hypnosis for childbirth say much of the pain that women experience during delivery comes from the expectation of pain, and the fear and tensions that this produces. They point out that in some cultures, where childbirth is not regarded as something to be fearful about, women experience less pain than women in western society. Prebirth sessions will focus on changing the mother's preconceptions as to what childbirth will involve. The aim is to get the mother's body working in harmony with the delivery to make it as stress-free as possible.

Often the mothers-to-be first undergo hypnosis sessions weeks before the expected birth in order to reframe their views of childbirth. They are then taught a variety of self-hypnosis techniques to use during the birth itself. It is important that the woman should become confident in her ability to use these techniques, a belief that can itself be strengthened by the hypnotist in the earlier sessions. Sometimes a therapist will make tapes for the mother to play during her labor, or will even be present herself.

The mother is encouraged in delivery to think of the natural pains as pressures or surges, rather than to use pain-associated expressions such as "contractions."

To be most successful, hypnosis should be employed as early as possible in the pregnancy. This not only helps to ensure that the woman is well used to the beneficial effects of hypnosis, but also means that the technique can be used to offset issues encountered early on, such as nausea, anxiety, and tiredness. It is also important that the woman seeks expert medical care alongside hypnosis to ensure the well-being of herself and her child. The evidence shows, however, that giving birth using hypnosis may be the answer to many women's prayers.

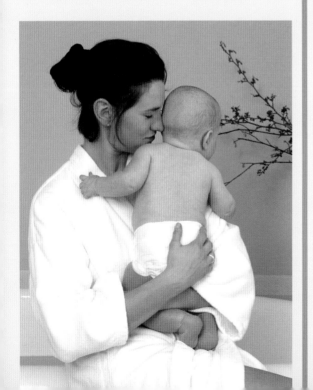

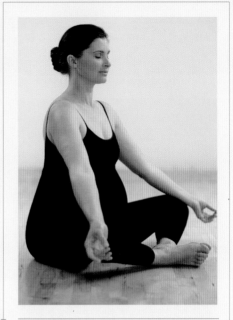

⌣Hypnosis does not just help with the actual birth, but with pregnancy, too. The positive experiences from hypnosis a woman enjoys while carrying the baby can help strengthen the effects of the treatment during birth itself.

Giving Birth under Hypnosis

Tania Lapointe gave birth to the third of her three children using hypnosis. Her first two births—to Guille and Philip—had been painful. "I was in extreme pain, the kind of pain where I was almost convulsing, screaming, 'Give me drugs, give me drugs,'" she said. For her third pregnancy, with her daughter Chlo, Tania underwent hypnosis at the HypnoBirthing Institute in New Hampshire, learned self-hypnosis techniques, and gave birth calmly and without any medication. The verdict? "This was like heaven compared to the other two," Tania told ABC News in May 2002. The woman who taught Tania, Maureen Saba, said, "Some of the basics are learning how to breathe properly, how to let the muscles completely relax. It really must be practiced at home. Self-hypnosis gets better with practice."

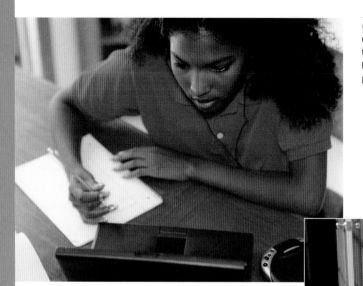

From the moment he or she is born, a child is undergoing a form of programming from experiences and people around him or her; using hypnosis can help shape that programming in a positive way.

Helping children

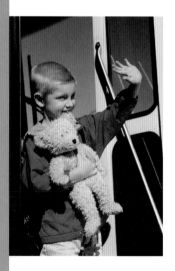

Children can be very good hypnotic subjects as they naturally accept the power of the imagination, the key to helping unlock the power of the unconscious mind.

It is well known that children tend to have more vivid imaginations than adults. This is why they often make better hypnotic subjects. Their young minds are more open to suggestions, free from the conscious doubts that adults tend to acquire over the years.

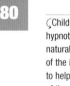

If adults are, in part, the sum of all the impressions, sensations, ideas that they have experienced throughout their lives, then a child is daily undergoing this process of programming. The views of a child's friends, teachers, and, above all, parents are shaping the child's view of the world. To a certain extent, children are seeing the world through their parents' eyes, and this inevitably helps mold the kind of person they become. Most of us will have experienced this phenomenon in relation to our teachers. It is quite common, later in life, to acknowledge how much our view of the world or about certain subjects was influenced by one or two memorable teachers. In the same way, teachers and parents can unwittingly be negative influences on children. Tell children often enough that they are "stupid" and the chances are that, deep down, they will begin to believe it. Or tell them enough that they are able to tackle any new challenges that come their way and pretty soon they will begin to think the same.

This means, of course, that hypnosis, and the use of suggestion, can be a very powerful tool for developing the behavior of children.

Hypnosis can be used to instill confidence in shy children and concentration in those who find it hard to focus on anything for more than a few seconds. It can be used to help learning and social skills, and to reduce anxiety.

More specifically, hypnosis sessions have been shown to be effective in dealing with childhood problems such as bed wetting, thumb sucking, recurring nightmares, nail biting, and stuttering. Other possible uses are for conditions such as dyslexia and obsessive-compulsive behavior. As with adults, it seems that for hypnosis to be effective a child has to want to change and work with the therapist, or at least not to oppose the therapy.

Though children generally have a shorter attention span than adults, they readily go into hypnosis; although, unlike most adults, they may often wriggle during a trance. In fact, so rich are children's imaginations that sometimes the hypnotist may not need to use a formal induction. When an induction technique is used, it will often focus on the child's strong imagination and special interests, perhaps a favorite book, television show, or movie. Very often children will be asked to visualize their heroes, either real ones or fictional characters such as Spiderman or Batman, to help solve their problems. Typically, most children do not remember what they were told during a hypnotic trance.

Naturally enough, many parents are nervous at leaving their children in the hands of a stranger who is going to "influence their minds." The solution is for parents, especially those with young children, to attend the sessions too. This also has the added benefit that the parents can then see for themselves the effectiveness of hypnosis.

Hypnosis is not usually performed on very young children, up to the ages of three or four. As they get older, kids can also be taught to use self-hypnosis.

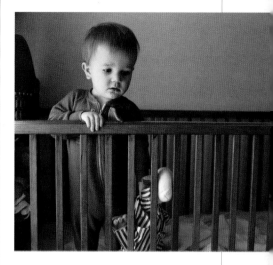

Monster Spray

A child often woke up crying because of a bad nightmare he constantly experienced involving monsters. His parents took him to a hypnotist, who talked to the boy. Together, and with the child in a trance, they created the idea of a "Monster Spray," which they would keep in a bottle with its own label. In this story the special spray was used to remove all the monsters from the child's house. After that the hypnotist created a shield that surrounded the child's house and room so that the monsters could never return. After just two sessions of this treatment, the boy's monster nightmares had vanished. This shows how vivid imagery, to which the child can relate, is often effective in hypnosis in implanting suggestions in children.

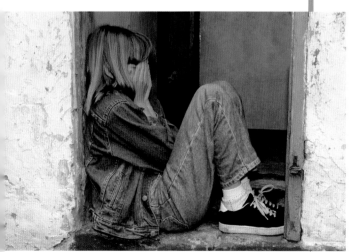

⌣Hypnotherapy can be useful in helping children who are suffering from low esteem or undue anxiety.

Enabling memory and learning

As well as medical and therapeutic uses, hypnosis has many other practical applications. One of these is in helping people study and then remember details. For many people, studying can be a problem. We get restless, find it hard to concentrate, and would rather be outside—anywhere—than stuck with our books. Then, when we do finally get down to some serious work, we discover within a few minutes that we are immediately forgetting everything we try to absorb.

Hypnosis is commonly used to deal with this problem in a number of ways. First, a hypnotist can get someone in the right frame of mind to start her studies. It doesn't matter what age she is or what subject she is studying, just as long as she has a desire to learn. The skilled hypnotist will draw on the student's own learning style—everyone has one—and build upon that. In a trance, the student will be told that she will be relaxed, calm, and ready to learn. She will be told that she will be able to remember what she learns, and understand its meaning.

The next step will be the examinations or tests that the student has to take. One of the biggest problems for students facing a test is an attack of nerves. It is a familiar feeling. The student has done hours of study, and knows her subject backward and forward, but, when faced with a blank sheet of paper in the test, the mind also seems blank. Panic then sets in, and it becomes nearly impossible to remember anything about the subject at all. Hypnosis

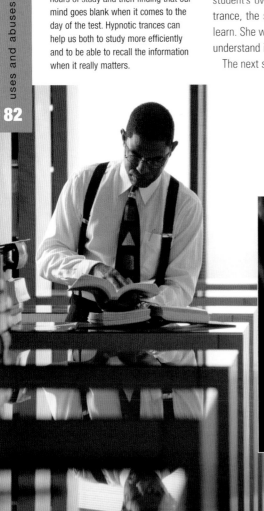

⌒There is nothing worse than doing hours of study and then finding that our mind goes blank when it comes to the day of the test. Hypnotic trances can help us both to study more efficiently and to be able to recall the information when it really matters.

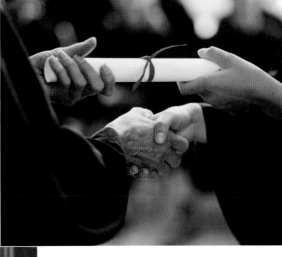

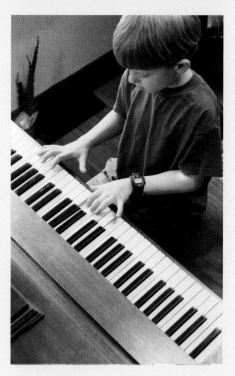

⟩We learn so many skills in our lives that later get forgotten, hidden in our minds. With hypnosis we can often unlock our minds and rediscover past skills such as playing the piano or speaking a foreign language.

can help overcome this common experience. Before the exam the student will undergo a number of hypnotic sessions. During these the therapist will suggest to the client's unconscious mind that at the time of the test she will feel calm, relaxed, and in full control of her thought processes. Her mind will feel alert and, above all, she will be able to remember in great detail all she has studied. It may also be suggested that after the test the student will feel calm and satisfied that she has done her best; this can help prevent post-test panic attacks. Getting the right results in tests is so important that anyone who suffers from nerves or panic attacks during them should consider trying hypnosis. It really does seem to work. Remember, though, that hypnosis will not help you pass your tests all by itself; you have to put the work in to make it happen.

Hypnosis can also apparently retrieve lost skills from the mind. There are anecdotes that suggest that people who once spoke a foreign language when they were young but have since forgotten it can recover the skill during a trance and afterward.

Another use of hypnosis is to help people learn speed-reading. Using hypnosis and speed-reading techniques, students can often at least double the speed at which they read and absorb—and also successfully retain—information.

A little-known use of hypnosis is as a research tool in other areas of science. Researchers put subjects into a trance and replicate natural phenomena such as alcohol intoxication so that they can study the state.

Forgotten Language

A woman named Ana had been brought up in India, where she spoke Punjabi, but had since moved to the West and spoke fluent English. Ana was still in touch with old friends from India but they communicated through a mixture of Punjabi and English, as she had forgotten much of her old language. A friend who was also a clinical hypnotist suggested to her that he put her into a trance to see if they could recover the lost language. Under hypnosis, the hypnotist, who did not know a word of the language himself, simply suggested that she could now speak Punjabi as well as ever. When Ana next spoke to her friends, she and they were both amazed to find that she could speak Punjabi fluently again. Using hypnosis to retrieve languages seems to be most successful if people absorbed them in the very early years of their lives, for the brain adapts to the patterns of language and this can then stay with people for the rest of their lives.

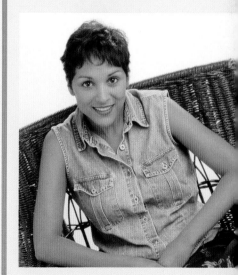

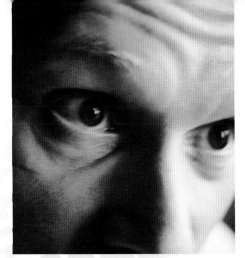

⟩The various techniques of age-regression therapy and past-life regression are among the most controversial in hypnosis as well as being the most fascinating. How accurately do we retain knowledge of all that has happened to us?

Regression and progression therapy

The technique of age regression and regression therapy is the most controversial in the whole field of hypnosis. It is also one of the most intriguing. The simple form of age regression is where a hypnotist induces a patient into a trance, and then takes that patient back into his past. Much more controversial, and hotly debated, is what is called past-life regression, where the patient is taken back to what seem to be previous lives. More bizarre still is the claim by some hypnotists that they can take subjects back to periods of existence between lives. As if that were not enough, some people have been taken forward in time, to what seems to be a future life, in so-called age progression.

Proponents of these techniques say that they are not just interesting experiences, but that they can be powerful healing tools as well. However, many experts are very skeptical about the nature of these "memories."

Age Regression

The use of hypnotic trance to take someone back into childhood has attracted bad publicity in recent years because of the so-called false-memory syndrome (see page 94). These were cases in which people under hypnosis "relived" apparent abuse in their childhood but were later found not to have experienced any abuse at all. This has raised serious question marks about the accuracy of any trance-induced recollections of the past. This is of huge importance when the recollections are intended to be used as possible evidence in a criminal trial or in scientific research.

However, age regression is still commonly used by hypnotists in treating patients. For therapy, it does not matter whether the remembered events

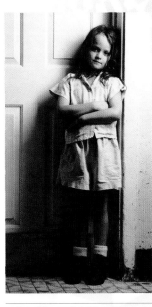

↶One of the most controversial aspects of regression therapy, often, but not always using hypnosis, is what is known as false-memory syndrome. This is where people appear to recall past events in their lives—such as abuse—which they have not in fact experienced.

actually took place; what really matters is whether the events are real to that person's unconscious mind. They are stories or metaphors, and therapists do not take them at face value. Our unconscious minds contain countless memories as well as a powerful imagination, and sometimes the two can get confused. We are all used to the experience of casting our minds back to recall an event, and not being quite sure whether it happened, or whether we have simply imagined that it happened. This does not matter to the unconscious mind, which behaves as if it did happen. These memories/imaginings work as symbolic stories that influence our unconscious mind's view of the world.

Hypnotists who use age regression as therapy believe that confronting past traumas or reawakening lost emotions can be of enormous benefit to patients. The memories are not taken literally; they are metaphors for the mind that have a specific meaning to the individual. The idea is that when patients connect their problems—they might be phobias, for instance—with the trigger cause in their childhood, the problems can disappear. Hypnotherapists call this process crossing the "affect bridge."

Age-regression therapy is used to treat a number of conditions, including phobias, deep-seated emotional problems, and relationship issues. In one example, a middle-aged woman named Alice had an inexplicable fear of water and had no idea what caused it. Under regression therapy, Alice was asked by her therapist to go back in her life until the first moment she had experienced her fear. She recalled that, when she was a very young child, an older brother had once thrown her into a swimming pool and it had caused her deep distress. The hypnotist encouraged Alice to recall what she felt about water before this event—she had liked it—and suggested that this was what she really felt now. Gradually, she overcame her fear of water and started to learn to swim.

Sometimes, just knowing what the trigger event was seems to help a person to overcome its effects; in other cases the hypnotist will need to work slowly with the patient while he or she comes to terms with it.

The Affect Bridge

The so-called "affect bridge" is an important tool in age-regression therapy. This is a technique where a patient under a trance is encouraged to make a connection in his mind between an event long ago that triggered a certain reaction/feeling in him—known as an "initial sensitizing event" (ISE)—and the resulting reaction/feeling that persists in him now. He uses his current mood as a metaphoric bridge to go back to when that mood was present before, including for the first time. The patient is encouraged to see that his old experience belongs to that past time, not to his current state. Sometimes the simple fact of making this connection can be enough to ease or remove the patient's problem.

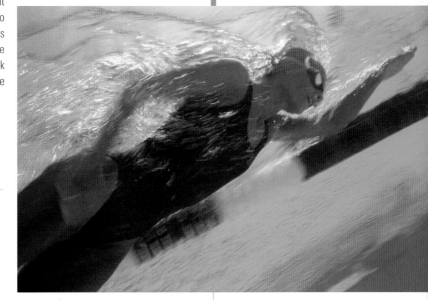

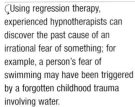

Using regression therapy, experienced hypnotherapists can discover the past cause of an irrational fear of something; for example, a person's fear of swimming may have been triggered by a forgotten childhood trauma involving water.

Past-Life Regression

This is still a very controversial area. For one thing, the idea that people have had previous lives—reincarnation—is at odds with the beliefs of many people with religious convictions and those with none. Most Christians, for example, do not now believe in the doctrine of reincarnation, though it was a widely accepted part of Christian belief for several centuries. What is curious, however, is that even people who do not believe in past lives do seem to experience them under past-life regression (PLR). Whether these are real experiences or not is bitterly disputed. Many scientists are adamant that these recollections are simply a cocktail of imagination, false memories, and possibly unintentionally implanted suggestions. Proponents of past-life experiences claim that many of the specific details of apparent past lives recalled under PLR can be explained only by the theory that those lives were real. Most people, however, including many hypnotists, simply do not know what to make of this strange phenomenon.

Some examples, such as where someone recalls he was a famous person, an Egyptian high priest, or a great warrior, may indeed be simply the imagination masquerading as memory. But many past lives are so mundane that one wonders where the inspiration for them comes from. Also, some of the information obtained is so obscure that its source cannot be easily identified. For the time being, such details remain unexplained.

Even patients who do not believe in past-life regression—when we are supposedly taken back to a previous life—experience this phenomenon while in trance. Quite what causes it is a controversial subject. Recalling an exotic life as an Egyptian high priest, Greek soldier, or famous person may be the result of cultural programming masquerading as memory.

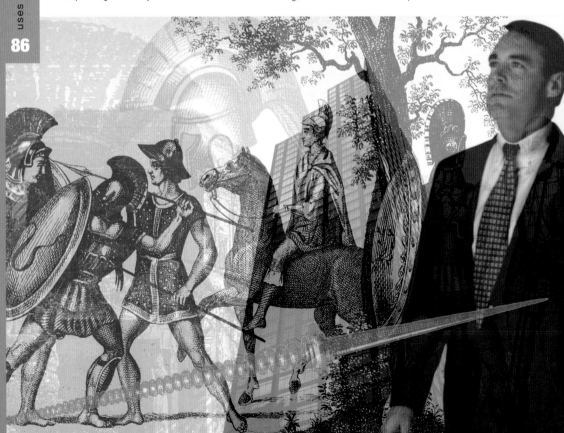

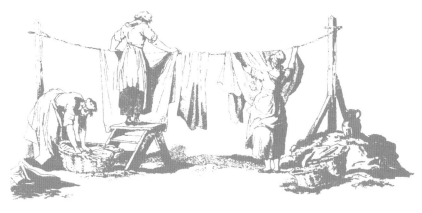

ꙅSome patients' past-life regression experiences are so mundane that one wonders what the inspiration for them is; in one example a man recalled living on an eighteenth-century landed estate in England. In another a man "remembered" a past life as a laundry woman. Could they be real?

However, PLR does have therapeutic value. Hypnotists who use PLR as therapy point out that, as with age regression, the experiences or stories "remembered" from past lives work as metaphors for the unconscious mind. They tell a story that is important to the mind and that can then be used by the hypnotist as a starting point for therapy.

The strangest PLR claims—and championed by a very few hypnotists—are that patients can be taken back to those periods after one life ends and before another starts, in effect, the spirit world. The ultimate form of this is taking the person back even further into his or her past, to the time before he or she had any incarnations at all, before time for them as a person started.

Age Progression

This is a technique that hypnotists sometimes use to help patients visualize how they can improve themselves by changing their behavior. For example, a person who knows she ought to give up smoking but doesn't really yet have the resolve to do so may be asked to imagine two different futures for herself. One will be of her still as a smoker in ten years' time, the other as a nonsmoker. The powerful image of the difference in the two lives is intended to persuade the smoker that she really wants to give it up now.

A more unusual age-progression technique is to take a patient beyond this life into her next life. This method, of course, raises many of the same ethical objections as past-life regression. In one recent case a professional man in London was progressed under deep trance by a clinical hypnotist into a future life. The good news was that in his next life he also lived in London. The less good news, for him, was that in this existence he was a road sweeper.

Past Lives

The past lives apparently recalled by hypnotic subjects can be quite mundane. In one recent case, a man recalled one life in which he had been working on the grounds of an estate in eighteenth-century England. In another life he had worked as a laundry woman. However, in a more celebrated case, the hypnotherapist Arnall Bloxham hypnotized a woman named Jane Evans and obtained detailed accounts of six previous lives over the past two millennia: as a tutor's wife in Roman times; as one of the many Jews who were massacred in twelfth-century England at York; as the servant of a French medieval merchant prince; as a maid of honor to Catherine of Aragon; as a poor servant in London during the reign of Queen Anne; and as a nun in nineteenth-century America. This is an exotic collection indeed. Critics claim most if not all memories of so-called past lives can be explained by the impact of the imagination and the remarkable ability of the mind to fabricate narrative from fragments of information. Supporters insist that not all cases can be explained in this way.

Winning at sports

We have all heard the sportsmen and the commentators say it. Winning, they say, is all in the mind. And they tap the side of their forehead with their finger to emphasize the point. So it should not be that surprising that hypnosis is increasingly widely used in sports to improve performances at all levels. After all, between two evenly matched teams or individuals, it is often the players who *really* believe they can win who come out on top.

What perhaps is surprising is how long it has taken some sportsmen and women to recognize the true value of hypnosis.

Take the example of Bob Reese, a former trainer with the New York Jets. He now runs his own company, which helps sportspeople, among others, to improve their performances. Reese learned early on that when he uses hypnotherapy in the hard-bitten arena of sports, it helps to give the technique a different name. He commented, "There was a built-in fear—they didn't want to give up their minds. Instead I started telling athletes we were going to do some high-powered visualization techniques."

Nowadays, that mistrust of hypnosis is beginning to soften, even within professional sport, and many leading sportspeople have used hypnotherapy. After all, there is increasing evidence that it works and no professional sports performer can afford to neglect a chance to boost his or her chances of winning.

For example, a scientific study was carried out in the United States involving 12 male and 12 female college basketball players over a season. The research showed that those who were hypnotized had better shooting averages than those in the group who had not undergone the hypnosis.

Those who inhabit the hard-bitten world of sport can be suspicious of new concepts; when former New York Jets trainer Bob Reese used hypnosis with players he found it best to use a different name to describe it.

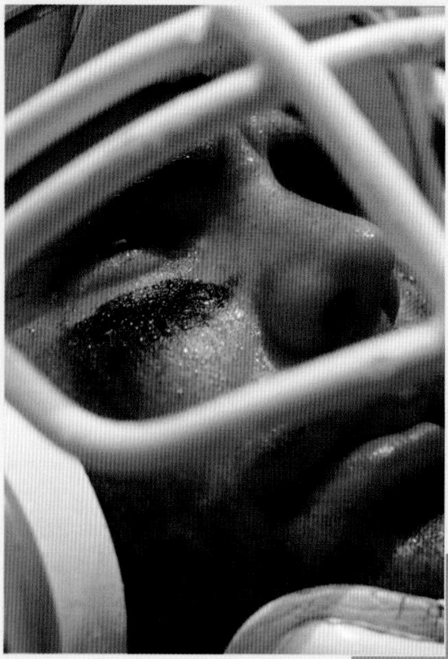

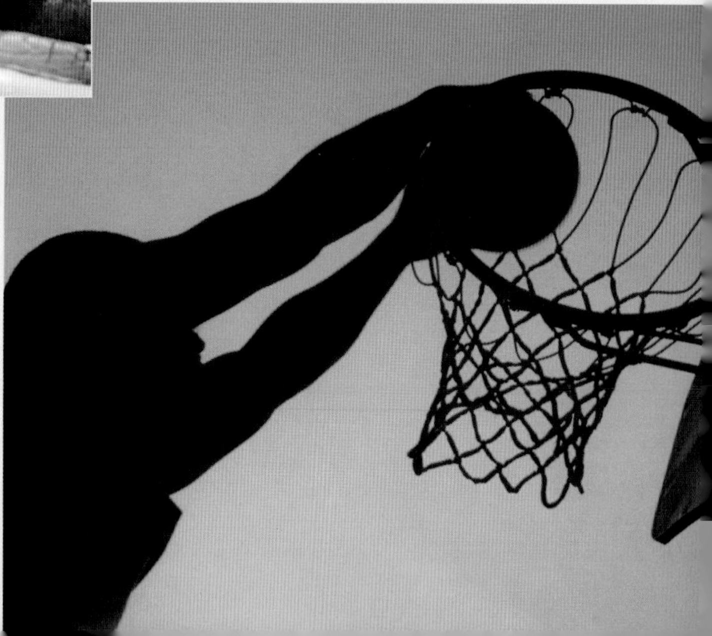

There is scientific evidence that hypnosis really can boost a player's or a team's performance. A study of college basketball players found that those who had undergone hypnosis had better shooting records than those who did not.

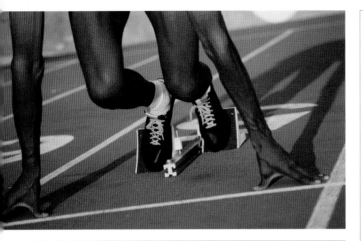

⤸The power of the mind has been shown in a remarkable scientific study of athletes. It was found that when the athletes visualized or imagined themselves performing their sport, a physical change took place in the muscles they would need to carry out those actions. It is this power of the mind that hypnosis unleashes.

Scientists have also shown something quite remarkable about the power of imagination. When athletes visualize or imagine themselves carrying out a performance, a change takes place in those muscles that would have been used had they really carried out that activity. There can be little better proof of the untapped resources of the human mind, which is precisely what is used during hypnosis.

Though they are used in team sports as well, hypnotherapy and visualization techniques are particularly common in individual sports or in team sports where there are individual one-on-one battles, such as baseball. Golf is one sport where hypnosis is especially common. Britain's Nick Faldo, one of the greatest golfers of the past two decades, and three times winner of the U.S. Masters, used a hypnotist. Even the great Tiger Woods uses visualization techniques that have been developed from hypnotism. Meanwhile, more and more amateur golfers of all levels are using self-hypnosis tapes or sessions with hypnotherapists to improve their game (see page 91).

Kurt Angle

The popular WWF wrestler and former Olympic champion Kurt Angle used hypnosis to reach the top in his sport. It started when Angle was training for the 1995 freestyle world championships at a gym in Pittsburgh. A fellow gym user, Andrew Yasko, was a police officer and also a hypnotist. Yasko persuaded his new friend that he could help the wrestler win the gold at both that event and the 1996 Olympics.

"I really didn't think hypnosis was going to work," says Angle, "but I was willing to try." After some 50 hypnosis sessions, in which Yasko told the wrestler's subconscious mind that he needed to be more focused and aggressive, Angle won gold in both titles. He readily acknowledges his debt to hypnosis in helping him achieve both goals. "It definitely worked even though I was skeptical at first," says Angle. "If you are a competitive athlete you need to be as mentally fit as you are physically. The human mind is so powerful. This was a completely natural, healthy way to get my mind ready for competition."

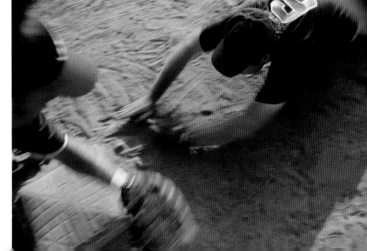

⤸Hypnosis is especially common in those sports involving individuals, or where the sport has individual one-on-one battles—such as baseball.

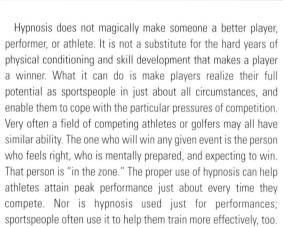

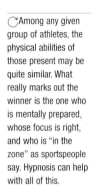

Among any given group of athletes, the physical abilities of those present may be quite similar. What really marks out the winner is the one who is mentally prepared, whose focus is right, and who is "in the zone" as sportspeople say. Hypnosis can help with all of this.

Hypnosis does not magically make someone a better player, performer, or athlete. It is not a substitute for the hard years of physical conditioning and skill development that makes a player a winner. What it can do is make players realize their full potential as sportspeople in just about all circumstances, and enable them to cope with the particular pressures of competition. Very often a field of competing athletes or golfers may all have similar ability. The one who will win any given event is the person who feels right, who is mentally prepared, and expecting to win. That person is "in the zone." The proper use of hypnosis can help athletes attain peak performance just about every time they compete. Nor is hypnosis used just for performances; sportspeople often use it to help them train more effectively, too.

One American athlete who has used hypnosis is Adam Heidt, a member of the U.S. Olympic luge team. Heidt has a trigger word—"assail"—which he uses if he gets too nervous before a run. This helps him stay calm and focused before the start.

Another example is the British athlete Iwan Thomas, a top 400-meter runner. Thomas had trouble blocking out the noise of the crowd and the activities of his opponents in big races. So he sought out a hypnotist, Robert Farago, who used exercises to help him concentrate. Before a big race, Thomas gently tugs on his left earlobe, a signal for him to go into a trance and focus on his own performance rather than on what anyone else is doing. It worked: in 1998 he won the World Cup title for the 400-meter event.

Often the sports hypnotist will focus on getting the athlete to learn how to compete against herself rather than against others. This puts the emphasis on her own performance, not on worrying what others will do, which can induce negative thoughts.

Some hypnotists say they can even spot who is likely to win a sporting contest before the start. They can tell those athletes who are focused and "in the zone," and those who subconsciously fall into step behind the ones who, deep down, they think will win. Sports truly are, as they say, all in the mind.

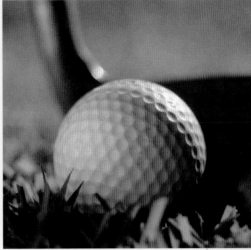

ςThey say sport is all in the mind; and some experienced sports hypnotists say they can tell who is going to win even before the game or contest, from observing who is most focused.

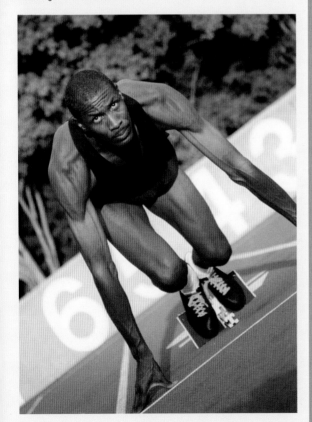

Golf and Hypnosis

Hypnosis is widely used by golfers to improve their game, as can be seen by the huge number of CDs, tapes, videos, and "hypno-golf" sessions available on the market. The technique is popular not just among the professionals, though many do use it, but among weekend players and amateurs, too. The reason for this is perhaps that golf is a very mental sport. Golfers are constantly battling not just against the course and conditions, but against themselves, too. Under pressure, the swing or the putt easily falls apart. Many players have, for example, experienced the dreaded "yips" in putting, when the hands seem to move all on their own and become out of control during the stroke. Under hypnosis, a player can learn how to overcome his inner hurdles. In a trance the golfer will visualize making the perfect swing, the perfect putt. He will learn to overcome the fears that cause tension, which in turn causes him to fluff his shots. The player learns how to recall the state of relaxation, calm, and mental strength he needs to play a shot. Hypnosis may not make you the next Tiger Woods, but it will ensure that you consistently play the best golf of which you are capable.

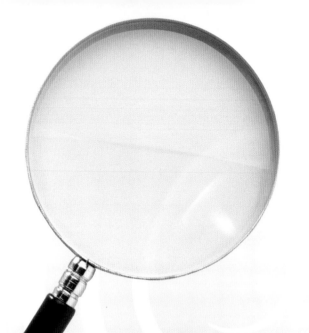

⌒The use of hypnotic trances to solve crimes and track down criminals has a long history. However, the use of the technique has been controversial, notably in the United States as courts cannot always be sure that the witness who recalls details of a crime has not been subtly influenced by his or her interrogators, or simply by his or her eagerness to help.

Forensic hypnosis

Anyone familiar with television crime shows or movies will know the age-old problem for the law-enforcement agencies: That witnesses often cannot remember much of what they witnessed. The details witnesses provide can be very few, even though they were present, and saw and heard everything. Forensic hypnosis—the application of hypnosis to solving crimes—is sometimes used to help in these situations.

The role of hypnosis in solving crimes has a long history. As long ago as 1845, a clairvoyant was put into a hypnotic trance to help identify a thief who had stolen a handful of dollars from a local store. Under hypnosis the woman described in detail a 14-year-old boy and said where he had gone when he had run out of the store. When he was apprehended, the youth was so amazed that he confessed to the crime on the spot.

Since the nineteenth century, however, the use of hypnosis in criminal investigations has been shrouded in controversy in the United States, as well as in other countries. The problem is that while witnesses and victims of crime may, under hypnosis, remember crucial details, how can anyone be sure these details are true? There is the question of what is called confabulation. This is the process in which the mind, perhaps aided by prompting, fills in the missing gaps in its memories with information that fits. The recall of this fabricated memory is not "lying" in the sense that it is intended to deceive, but it is invented. This problem is compounded by the fact that investigators may know what answers they want, and may consciously or unconsciously lead the witness or victim toward these answers. Similar issues have been identified in instances of so-called false-memory syndrome in alleged child-abuse cases (see page 94). The result has been a complex approach by different U.S. courts to the validity of evidence and testimony acquired under hypnosis.

In the notorious case of Ted Bundy in the late 1970s and early 1980s, the evidence of a witness produced under hypnosis was crucial to the prosecution's case that Bundy had abducted and murdered a 12-year-old girl, Kimberley Leach. The main witness could initially remember very few details, but in a trance recalled vital evidence that seemed to prove Bundy's guilt. On appeal, it was held that the court had been wrong to rely on this evidence, because the evidence produced under hypnosis did not tally with the evidence the witness had given earlier. As it happened, Bundy's petition was refused anyway and he later confessed to the murder of 28 women and was executed.

The use of evidence obtained under hypnosis varies in America from state to state. Moreover, there are clear guidelines as to how such evidence should be acquired: the hypnotist should not be regularly employed by the prosecuting authorities; the hypnotist should be genuinely expert; all interviews should be taped; and great care has to be taken not to lead the hypnotized witness toward particular answers.

Despite these problems and the complex legal situation, hypnosis continues to play a valuable part in solving crimes. In particular, it can be very useful in cases where there are few leads, no prime suspect, and where the investigators simply need to have more information on which to base their inquiries. That way, there is far less chance that the witness will, subconsciously, simply give the investigation team the answers it wants to hear. At such times, what witnesses recall under hypnosis can provide vital breakthroughs.

The Boston Strangler

In the infamous case of the Boston Strangler in the 1960s, a hypnotist was used to test whether Albert DeSalvo's dramatic confession to the 11 murders was genuine. At the request of the defense team, Dr. William J. Bryan Jr., from the American Institute of Hypnosis in Los Angeles, examined DeSalvo. Under hypnosis the defendant maintained his guilt and gave apparently convincing details of at least one of the murders, using information that probably only the killer could have known. This examination helped convince detectives that the confession was genuine. DeSalvo was in fact never tried on these charges, so the accuracy of the hypnotic confession was not put to the test. He was convicted for other offenses and was stabbed to death in prison in 1973. Since DeSalvo's death many have continued to claim that he was not actually the real Boston Strangler.

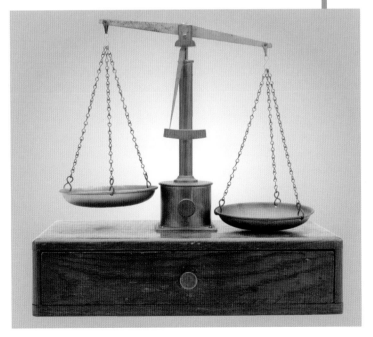

⌒Though hypnosis may have its limitations in solving crimes, especially in providing usable evidence, it can be very useful in cases where there are no prime suspects and where there are few leads. In such difficult cases, the witness may be able to recall valuable new information that may lead to a fresh line of inquiry; and there is also less risk of the investigator unwittingly influencing the witness toward a pre-determined outcome.

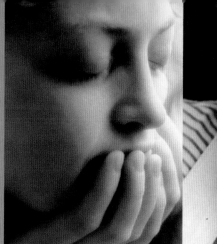
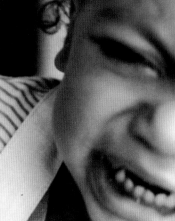

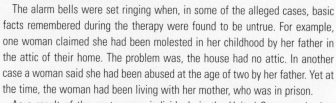
Hypnosis is one of the techniques used to help patients recall or recover forgotten traumas of the past, sometimes known as repressed or recovered memories. Often these memories may go right back to early childhood.

False-memory syndrome

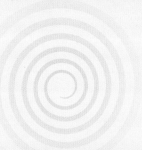

Hypnosis has become dragged into the bitter controversy over so-called false-memory syndrome. This involved cases where, in therapy, patients remembered events of abuse from their past that had hitherto remained forgotten. These are sometimes referred to as repressed or recovered memories. In fact, those "memories" often turned out to be false, and the alleged perpetrators were falsely accused. Not all of these cases have involved hypnosis. In some, other forms of therapy were used. However, the use of hypnosis in many of the controversial cases has thrown the spotlight on the technique and cast doubts on its ability to recover memories.

The alarm bells were set ringing when, in some of the alleged cases, basic facts remembered during the therapy were found to be untrue. For example, one woman claimed she had been molested in her childhood by her father in the attic of their home. The problem was, the house had no attic. In another case a woman said she had been abused at the age of two by her father. Yet at the time, the woman had been living with her mother, who was in prison.

As a result of the controversy, individuals in the United States and other countries found guilty of apparent abuse have had their cases overturned. Very often, the only real evidence of the abuse was from alleged victims, and they had recalled the relevant details only in therapy. One knock-on effect has been that some patients have later sued therapists for allegedly implanting these so-called false memories into their minds. The essential question is: How reliable are memories induced under hypnosis?

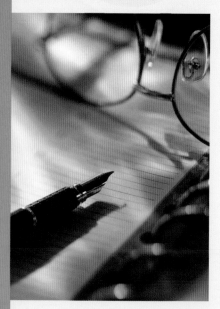

In therapy, patients may verbally recall errors, which the therapist commits to paper. These have sometimes led to false accusations of abuse, especially against parents.

Back in 1985, a statement from the Council on Scientific Affairs of the American Medical Association warned that "recollections obtained during hypnosis can involve confabulations and pseudo-memories and not only fail to be more accurate, but actually appear to be less reliable than nonhypnotic recall."

Confabulation is where a person gives false or contrived answers to questions about the past, believing the answers to be true, filling in the gaps of lost memory. More recently, in 1993, the American Psychiatric Association warned that repressed memories could be false, particularly when therapists were involved in the recovery of these memories.

These warnings came at a time when many families in the United States and elsewhere were being torn apart by allegations of abuse. Some of the worst cases included claims of ritual satanic abuse, and the atmosphere at the time has been likened to the witch-hunt hysteria of the sixteenth and seventeenth centuries, including that at Salem, Massachusetts, in 1692. As a result of the outcry, the False Memory Syndrome Foundation was founded in Philadelphia and similar bodies were established in other parts of the world.

Critics point out that such recovered "memories" are sometimes the fault of therapists who are hunting for repressed memories of childhood abuse, and who continue until they find them. In such circumstances and under this pressure, the unconscious mind, which is open to suggestion and the power of imagination, may end up supplying such details simply to please the interrogator. Once these memories have been created, they become as real as any other memory and acquire the status of truth in the mind of the patient. A further problem is that some therapists have diagnosed (often incorrectly) their patients with multiple-personality disorder (MPD)—now known as dissociative-identity disorder (DID)—for which they assumed childhood abuse was the cause. This made them even more determined to unlock these missing memories in the patient's mind. Many experts, in fact, now argue that incidents of serious and genuine child abuse are rarely completely forgotten by the victims, though they may be pushed to the back of the mind.

This does not mean that all memories recalled under hypnosis are false, or that hypnotherapy in which patients are encouraged to go back to their childhood does not help them. However, it does mean that recovered memories of apparent past criminal acts are unlikely to be the basis of legal action unless there is very strong external supporting evidence for them.

The Eileen Franklin case

The most notorious criminal case involving apparent repressed memory was that of Eileen Franklin and her father George from California. Undergoing therapy during 1989 and 1990, Eileen began to recall details of the murder of her best friend, Susan Nason, who had been killed twenty years before. Eileen now said that it was her father who had first raped, then killed the girl. Based on this evidence, George Franklin was convicted of murder. His daughter also "remembered" his killing another woman in 1976. Although at the time Eileen had denied recalling this information under hypnosis, her sister later testified that both girls had been under hypnosis when recalling the details of the past. It later emerged that DNA evidence proved that George Franklin could not have been the killer in the 1976 case, for which he also had a strong alibi. There was also evidence suggesting that Eileen's belated recall of the 1969 killing was based on media reports at the time, including errors contained in those accounts. In 1996 all charges were dropped and Franklin walked free.

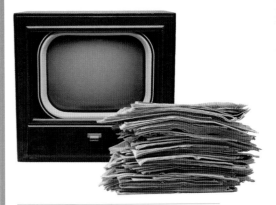

∿The case of Eileen Franklin in the United States underlines the potential pitfalls of relying solely on apparently repressed memory. Under therapy, Eileen "recalled" that her father George had killed a girl back in 1969, and also a woman in 1976. Yet forensic evidence proved that he could not have committed the 1976 killing, and eventually all criminal charges against him were dropped.

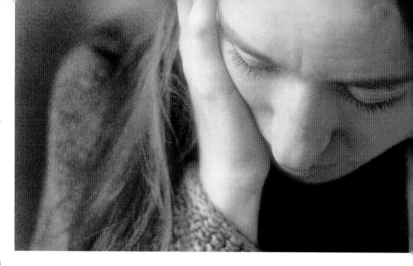

◯A few headline-grabbing cases of abuse perpetrated by hypnotherapists against their patients have raised concern about the dangers of the therapy. Yet there is no evidence that hypnotherapists are any more likely to abuse their patients than other medical practitioners such as doctors and dentists; all such cases are mercifully rare.

Abuse of patients

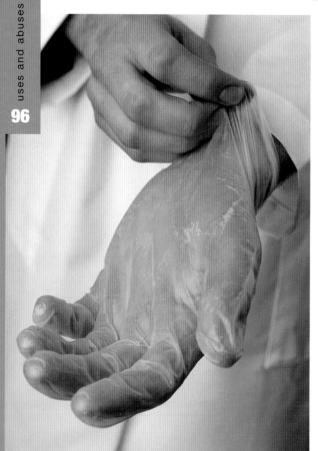

The bond between hypnotherapist and patient is the same as any relationship between therapist and client—it relies on mutual trust. In the overwhelming majority of cases the hypnotist goes to extraordinary lengths to win and maintain this trust and to work to the standard ethical levels of any healing practitioner. Just occasionally, however, and as has been the case with doctors, dentists, surgeons, and counselors, the relationship has been abused. There is no evidence that hypnotists are more likely to break this trust than anyone else, and most of the cases have involved an abuse of the healer-patient trust inherent in any medical relationship rather than a misuse of the trance state itself. However, the public's perception that hypnosis could be used on someone against his or her will—and knowledge—makes this a particularly sensitive issue.

There certainly have been cases in the United States, and elsewhere, of hypnotists being accused of using hypnotism to assault or have sex with a patient. These cases raise an important point about whether it is possible to have sex with someone under hypnosis without his or her consent or even knowledge. This debate has a long history. In 1865 in France there was a well-publicized case of a tramp called Timothée, who had a reputation as a magician and hypnotist. He was accused of abducting a 26-year-old woman, making her behave in various strange ways, and ultimately of raping her. During the court case, various experts were called as witnesses and they testified that it was indeed possible for a hypnotist to have complete control over another person, as appeared to be the case here. Timothée was duly convicted of rape. Much more recently, in northwest England, a hypnotherapist was accused of raping a middle-aged client while she was under hypnosis. The man, who was aged 70, was acquitted after a jury heard that at the time of the alleged assaults he had been impotent. In another case, DNA tests showed that a gynecologist who had used hypnotism on a female patient was the father of her child, even though she was adamant that she could not remember the assault and would never have given consent to it (see opposite).

Many experts argue that it is not possible to have sex with people under hypnosis against their will. They insist that there is always a part of the mind that is aware of what is happening during a trance and that, if something like this happens to a person, he or she will come out of hypnosis. A recent survey in Britain, however, does indicate that abuse by hypnotherapists may in fact be underreported.

In one of the cases, given anonymously to a research group, a woman patient claimed she awoke from a trance to find her clothing undone, though she had no recollection that anything had happened. Her hypnotist merely remarked that sexual healing was very useful. Nor is the issue confined to sexual conduct. Another patient told the researchers that the hypnotherapist persuaded her to hand over large sums of money to him during the course of a number of sessions. Neither case gave rise to a formal complaint or went to court, so the allegations cannot be verified. There is still no evidence that abuses by hypnotherapists are any more common than those by other medical practitioners, which are rare.

Away from therapy, there is some disquiet about individuals and companies who produce cassettes, tapes, and seminars offering to tell men how to seduce any woman they want simply by using hypnosis. Though this is not illegal, most therapeutic hypnotists think that using hypnosis for this kind of end brings it into disrepute.

The British Gynecologist

In 2001 a British gynecologist, Darwish Hasan Darwish, was acquitted by a jury of raping a middle-aged woman who had been a patient many years earlier. The woman had undergone hypnosis to help her relax, and it emerged through DNA tests that her daughter was fathered by Darwish rather than by her husband. Under legal rules, the jury had not been told that Darwish, then 55, was already serving a six-year prison sentence for sexual assaults on a number of other female patients.

In a 1999 court hearing those victims had told how the doctor had hypnotized them into trances before sexually abusing them. These offenses had continued for ten years. They had not come forward to the authorities before because they felt their stories would not be believed. Even after the case, experts argued over whether it would have been possible for the woman in the later case to have been raped during hypnosis without her having any knowledge of it.

⤶In one anonymous survey of hypnotherapy patients, a woman claimed that during the course of a number of sessions she had been "persuaded" to hand over large sums of money to her therapist.

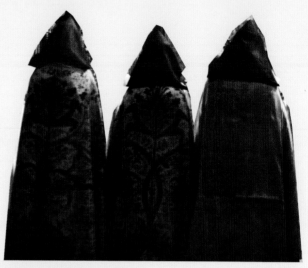

○Critics of hypnosis claim it can be used to make a person act against his or her will, for example to remain in cults—but the high dropout rate among such groups suggests that if the members do not like being a part of the cult they can, and do, choose to get out.

Cults, brainwashing, and mind control

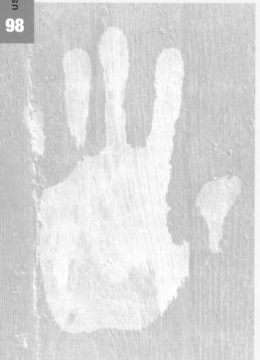

Do cults use hypnosis? The emergence of so many different cultlike groups in society has inevitably drawn attention to how they operate. They are often accused of splitting up families, and of influencing impressionable young people against their will and manipulating their behavior. Well-publicized tragedies such as the Jonestown massacre have only heightened such fears. On that occasion, in November 1978, the leader of the People's Temple cult, Jim Jones, ordered more than 900 of his followers to swallow a cyanide-laced drink at their base in Guyana. Guards were then ordered to shoot anyone who did not obey this terrible command.

Psychologists and sociologists argue over whether cults truly operate total "mind control" over their members. Those who doubt the mind-control theory say that while cults do use techniques to try to indoctrinate and control followers, these methods have their limitations and cannot alone completely control a person's thoughts and behaviors against his or her real wishes. This theory implies that for whatever reason, perhaps originally out of curiosity or a desire to seek something more in their lives, cult members are not operating entirely against their will. The evidence for this includes the fact that the dropout rate of many authoritarian cults is quite high as members become disillusioned and leave.

Experts who believe that such groups *do* exercise a form of mind control say that hypnosis is simply one of a number of techniques used to maintain authority over followers. They believe that members are put into a trance by methods including prolonged chanting, meditation, and the repetition of phrases. Once in a hypnotic trance, the subjects are open to suggestions made about the cult's beliefs to the unconscious mind.

The problem with this view, in relation to hypnosis, is that it conflicts with the theory that no one can be hypnotized against his or her will and that, once under hypnosis, a person cannot be made to do or believe anything that goes against his or her core values.

Few doubt that some cults do use forms of hypnosis with which they reinforce the cult's values, many of which are bizarre, fantastical, and often complete nonsense. Yet whether these groups use hypnotic techniques utterly to transform a person's personality against his or her real self is still very much open to doubt.

Brainwashing and Hypnosis

The word "brainwashing" was coined around 1950. The concept coincided with an era when the United States in particular was deeply concerned about the international spread of communism, following the end of World War II. Brainwashing is defined by *The Chambers Dictionary* as "the subjection of people to systematic indoctrination or mental pressure to make them change their views or confess to crimes etc." A rare phenomenon, it involves the complete transformation of the personality, usually after some kind of crisis or breakdown. Even then, the effects are usually temporary, unless continually reinforced. The word has now passed into everyday speech to refer to even the most harmless means by which we change our views on something. When it was first used, however, there was concern that brainwashing was being employed, specifically by communists, to influence a whole generation of people to totalitarian ideas. This was highlighted during the Korean War (1950–1953), when many U.S. servicemen were taken prisoners of war. The sight of thousands of American soldiers being paraded to denounce "imperial aggression" and offer support for communism convinced the authorities and the public that brainwashing was not just a theoretical threat, but a real and serious menace. Though drugs, deprivation techniques, and other methods were used as well, hypnotism was presumed to be one of the key ways in which the victims were being brainwashed. This meant that the U.S. authorities, and specifically the CIA, became fascinated with the idea of mind control and hypnosis in the 1950s and 1960s.

It is extremely doubtful that hypnosis can make someone reject his or her core moral or religious beliefs, or make him or her act in a way that conflicts directly with those beliefs.

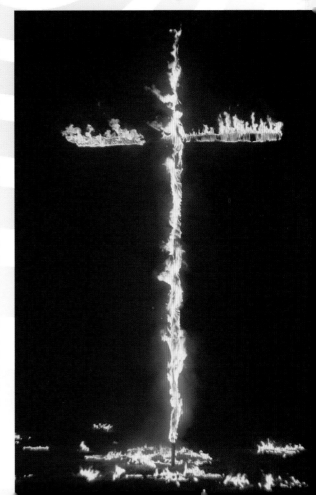

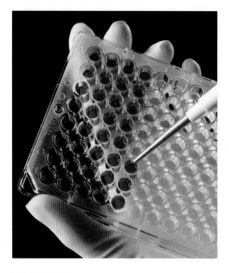

⤳German efforts to experiment with drugs and hypnotism during World War II met with little success.

The CIA and *The Manchurian Candidate*

During World War II, German scientists had experimented with using drugs and hypnotism on subjects to see if they could achieve mind control, but had limited success. An American government official, Stanley Lovell, had also discreetly consulted a number of renowned psychologists to see if hypnosis could be used in controlling individuals, only to be informed that it could not make people do things they would not normally do. For a while, the idea was dropped. One American professor of psychology, George Estabrooks, did believe hypnosis had military applications. These included the creation of hypnotized spies or hypnotizing captured spies for interrogation. He even wrote a book about it. But it was not until the late 1940s and early 1950s, with the Cold War well under way, that the potential military uses of hypnosis were properly explored.

In 1951 a senior CIA official, Morse Allen, was put in charge of the hypnosis project. Curious as it might sound, he had been impressed by the performance of a stage hypnotist, with whom he subsequently spent several days studying hypnotic techniques. In one later experiment Allen hypnotized a secretary and, using suggestion, induced her to fire a gun at a colleague. The gun was of course unloaded, but it seemed to prove that hypnosis could be used to make someone perform an act contrary to normal behavior. At about the same time, the CIA used a combination of drugs and hypnosis to interrogate two suspected Russian spies, including a posthypnotic suggestion that they later forget about the interrogation.

The ultimate goal, at least in the eyes of some military experts, was to create automaton assassins who would carry out a killing at a specific trigger or signal. This is the idea behind

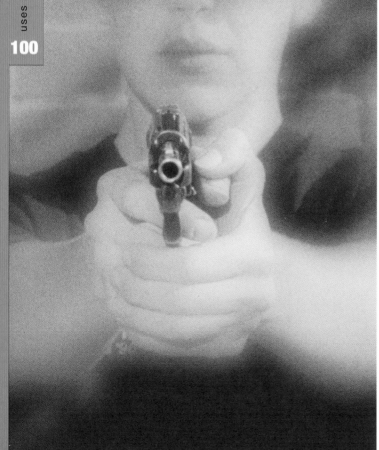

⤳The Central Intelligence Agency (CIA) was interested in hypnosis as a possible form of mind control. In one experiment official Morse Allen gave his hypnotized secretary a gun to fire at a colleague, which she did. Fortunately it was unloaded.

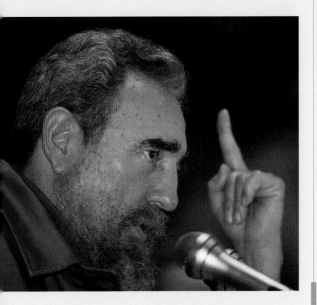

↪The unsuitability of hypnosis for producing reliable mind control in the field of espionage was underlined by a failed CIA plot to kill Cuban leader, Fidel Castro, using a hypnotized assassin.

the well-known book and later film *The Manchurian Candidate* (see box, this page).

Two attempts at hypnotic assassination are thought to have been tried, both in the 1960s. In one, a suspected double agent was to be hypnotized to kill his local KGB boss, but at the last minute the hypnotist refused to go along with the idea. In the other, a farfetched scheme to send a hypnotized Cuban exile over to Cuba to assassinate Fidel Castro fell through when, after three attempts, a suitable candidate could not be found.

Such failures began to convince the CIA that hypnosis had little use in their operations, except perhaps for interrogation. The fears of widespread brainwashing of American POWs also receded as it became clear that most of those who had apparently converted to communism in captivity had simply done so out of a very conscious, and quite understandable, sense of self-preservation.

Hypnosis was simply not an effective military tool. It could not be used on unwilling subjects or make people do what they really did not want to do. The case of the secretary who shot her colleague might seem to disprove this. However, she knew that it was her boss who was asking, that he was a government official, and that it was an experiment—and therefore presumably trusted that her employer would not make her do anything bad.

The Manchurian Candidate

The 1962 film *The Manchurian Candidate* was based on the thriller novel by Richard Condon, which had been written three years earlier. Both book and film appeared during the middle of the Cold War. The central character is an American soldier, Raymond Shaw, who is captured with others from his unit during the Korean War. Shaw (played in the film by Lawrence Harvey) and his friends (one played by Frank Sinatra) are hypnotized by a Chinese expert. They are returned to America at the end of the war, but by then Shaw has been turned into a hypnotized assassin, programmed to kill on behalf of the Chinese and Koreans. His trigger to kill is playing a game of solitaire—when the queen of diamonds comes up he goes into a passive state to receive instructions. Needless to say, Shaw, whose mother has remarried a virulently anticommunist senator, is completely unaware of his programming. This excellent thriller was removed from distribution after the assassination of President Kennedy a year later, but has now been reissued to renewed acclaim. Though its portrayal of hypnosis is flawed, the film brilliantly captures the fears over brainwashing and mind control by communist powers that existed during this period.

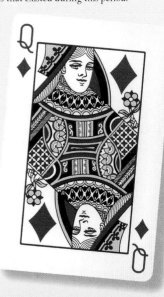

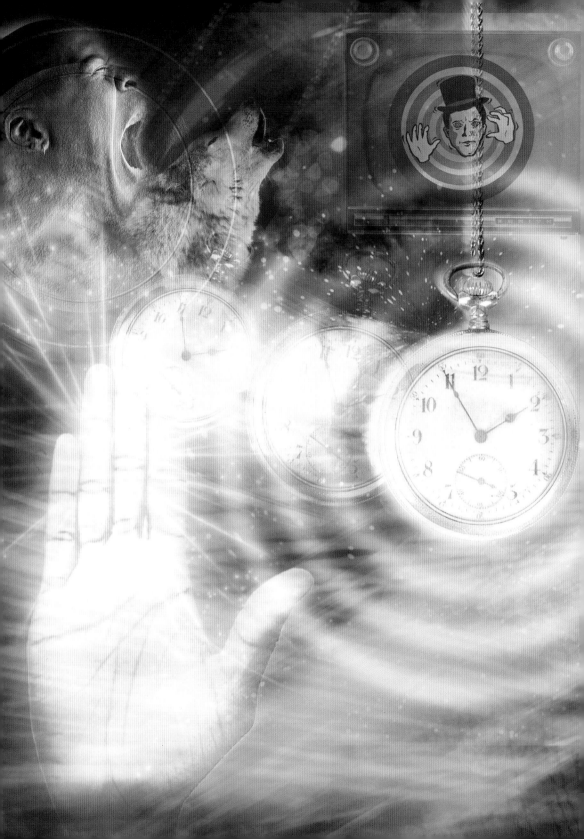

4: Stage Hypnosis

For many of us, our only contact with hypnosis is through entertainers—the colorful and exciting world of the stage hypnotist. Many of these are brilliantly talented hypnotists in their own right, and indeed, in the history of hypnosis, the stage performers of the past in America and Europe are often credited with keeping the technique alive. Sometimes, though, a stage act can go wrong and problems may occur. Some therapeutic hypnotists consider that their stage colleagues give hypnosis a bad name, in spite of the fact that many are accomplished therapists, too.

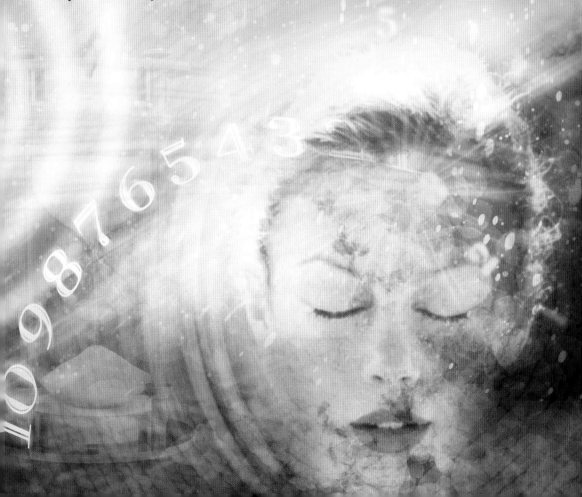

↪Stage hypnosis is a popular form of entertainment, whether on television or in live shows, and may be most people's sole experience of the phenomenon.

Show business

For many people, their only contact with hypnosis may be through the entertainment business—via stage hypnotists. Hypnotic entertainers have been around since the days of Mesmer in the eighteenth century and their popularity is as great as ever. Nowadays, hypnotic entertainers appear frequently on television shows as well as on tour with their stage productions or at fairs. These shows are usually very entertaining and the top performers in the United States and elsewhere have lucrative careers.

How does this use of hypnosis differ from the research and clinical applications discussed elsewhere in this book? Essentially, the techniques are broadly the same. A stage performer puts members of an audience into a hypnotic trance, bypasses the conscious mind, then uses the power of suggestion on the unconscious mind.

An Entertaining Audience

The key difference, of course, is that on stage or television all this is done purely for entertainment and not for therapy, so the kinds of suggestions a performer will put to a member of the audience will be very different from those used by a clinical hypnotist. Stage-show participants might be told to walk or quack like a duck, flap their "wings" like a bird, dance like a ballerina, confront "aliens," or swat at an imaginary fly. Or volunteers might believe that they have just won the U.S. Masters golf tournament, climbed a mountain, or just trashed their new Cadillac without insurance. There are countless different suggestions that stage hypnotists might put to their subjects, very few of which would be used in therapeutic work.

Another important difference is in the speed and depth of a trance. In therapy, the hypnotist will often take a while to induce a trance in the patient. Some individuals are less easy to hypnotize than others, and the therapist will establish which induction techniques are best for a particular client. The therapist will also perform quite a lot of work using a relatively light trance.

By contrast, the stage hypnotist has to work quickly. If he or she takes too long to guide someone gently into trance, the audience might soon be heading for the exits. Also, the entertainers usually put their subjects into a deep trance, so they can induce phenomena such as amnesia; therefore the stage hypnotist has to make sure that only the most hypnotizable members of the audience are used as participants.

This is why performers study their audiences very carefully, including during the warm-up. They will be looking for the signs that a person is particularly open to being hypnotized and might use suggestibility tests to see who responds best. Such tests might include asking members of the audience to close their eyes and imagine that one arm is attached to a balloon filled with helium. They are asked to imagine that the arm is getting lighter and lighter, until it starts moving upward, apparently without conscious effort. Anyone whose arm starts moving in such a test is likely to be a good candidate for hypnosis.

The performer will also be looking for a volunteer who shows interest in the subject of hypnosis and is a willing participant in the performance. Such enthusiasts are far more likely to make good stage-hypnotic subjects then someone who is skeptical or plainly unenthusiastic.

The need to select the most suitable members of the audience is also the reason why in shows you see a hypnotist choosing far more volunteers than he or she really needs for the act. This allows the performer to reject those who do not subsequently show they can easily be put into a deep trance. None of this happens by accident; stage hypnotists are taught the techniques of choosing the right subjects for hypnosis.

Acting Against Their Will?

This process of screening the audience should not be seen as in any way underhanded. The name of the game, after all, is entertainment, and the audience pays money to see people being hypnotized easily and then performing. They will not want the show to be taken up with the hypnotist slowly coaxing reluctant volunteers to take part. Choosing the right participants should therefore be seen as part of the skill of the performer.

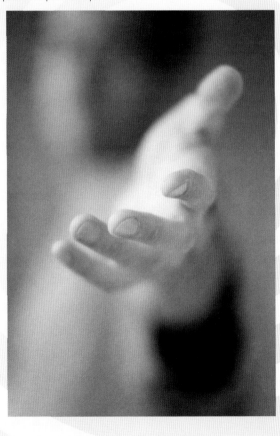

Part of the fun of stage hypnosis occurs when the performer invites volunteers up to be hypnotized to see what he or she can be "made" to do.

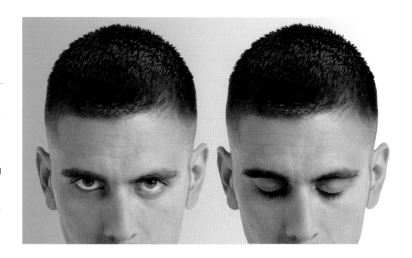

One of the trance-inducing techniques that a stage hypnotist will use on an audience volunteer is to suggest that his or her eyelids are getting heavier and heavier, and that he or she is finding it hard to keep his or her eyes open.

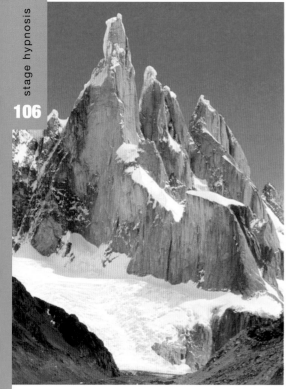

Suggestions to volunteers in stage shows will be very different than those used in therapeutic hypnosis sessions. Participants may believe they have just done something incredible—like climbing a mountain.

The selection process also helps answer one of the key questions raised about stage hypnosis—can they make the audience perform acts against its will, against what it believes in, or against what it would normally do? Most, though not all, hypnotists believe that people cannot be made to act against their will. So, in the case of stage shows, the fact that the audience participants are already anxious to take part in the show means that they have already agreed to go along with the act. It is true that in usual circumstances they might not normally run around a theater clucking like a chicken. But they have come to a show, they want to take part, and are therefore willing to have some fun in accordance with the nature of the routine.

The Stage Hypnotist

A good stage hypnotist is no less skilled at trance induction and suggestion than therapeutic practitioners, even if the techniques are used for different purposes. In bygone eras, it is true, fakes sometimes conned the audience into thinking they were putting people into a trance, when in fact the "volunteer" was a stooge of the performer. This no longer happens, because there are so many genuinely talented hypnotists around. Some are, in fact, brilliantly skilled, able to induce a deep trance very quickly and use suggestions swiftly and effectively. Moreover, a number of stage hypnotists have previously been therapists, others go on to become therapists, and some do both at the same time. So the gulf between those who perform stage hypnosis and those who use it for therapy is not as huge as it may seem.

However, stage hypnotists do have different requirements and priorities. First, they need to be good entertainers with stage presence. They have to enjoy performing. Also, they need to be quite dominant personalities, at least in their shows. In therapeutic hypnosis, the hypnotist and patient are a team, working together. On the stage, the performer is firmly in charge. The suggestions he or she might make are not of the permissive kind where the subject's mind is slowly guided in one direction. The stage performer uses direct, authoritarian suggestions: "You *will* quack like a duck."

The atmosphere of the show is also important. The stage hypnotist wants to encourage a group atmosphere, an excited expectation among the whole audience about what is going to happen. This helps get the volunteers in the mood, as they feel they are truly participating in the show. If the mood is right, the audience participants are already on their way to being hypnotized even before the formal induction process startss.

Skills of the Showman

Stage hypnotists do not have time on their side. They have to be able to induce a trance quickly in volunteers before the rest of the audience becomes bored. That is why they have to choose easily hypnotizable subjects who will respond to direct commands. One of the common techniques is to invite a large group of volunteers on stage, tell them to relax, and then inform them their eyelids are getting heavy and they can no longer keep them open. Those who respond well to this simple induction will stay; the others will be asked to leave the stage. A strong stage presence also helps, swiftly persuading people that the hypnotist is in charge. Often, stage hypnotists like to give the illusion that they are using magic powers to put people into a trance and then control them with suggestions. Such an approach adds to the likelihood that the volunteers will willingly go along with the induction, and achieve a deep trance rapidly. It is all part of the act. For example, some performers may use what are called "hand passes," whereby their energy is supposedly passed to the subject's body via the hypnotist's hands. This is an antiquated throwback to the days of mesmerism, but does add to the drama of the act. A key factor is stagecraft—setting the mood from the beginning. This will involve the right lighting, music, and a sense of drama from the start. Often the hypnotist will start with a volunteer who has been hypnotized before the show to demonstrate the "mystery of hypnosis." This increases the audience's belief in the hypnotist, which in turn will make it easier to hypnotize them.

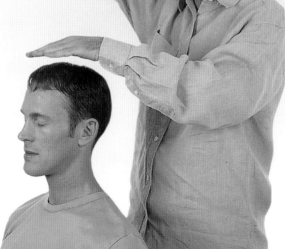

⌣The use of "hand passes" by a stage hypnotist is all part of the act; the hand movements are simply a visible device to help to create the belief that hypnosis is taking place.

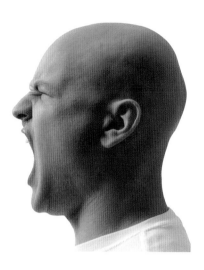

Questions and concerns

Ethical Doubts

The majority of people who go to watch stage hypnosis may think it is all good harmless entertainment, and very enjoyable at that. Yet many in the therapeutic world of hypnosis have deep reservations about stage hypnosis. Critics say that the shows bring hypnosis into disrepute by trivializing it and giving the general public a warped sense of what hypnosis really is, and by not emphasizing the many benefits it can bring. One of the first things hypnotherapists are often asked by new clients is whether they are going to be made to walk like a duck or cluck like a chicken or act out any of the other clichés of stage performance. Ultimately, the critics suggest, these unhelpful impressions could deter potential patients who would benefit greatly from hypnosis from seeking that help.

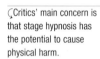

Critics' main concern is that stage hypnosis has the potential to cause physical harm.

Stage hypnotists counter this view by claiming that their shows can have precisely the opposite effect on people. By seeing firsthand the potential power of hypnosis on stage, they argue, members of the public are more likely to believe in the therapeutic effects of it. Whoever is right, hypnotic showmanship and therapeutic hypnosis have existed side by side for many decades, and this uneasy relationship is likely to continue for many years to come.

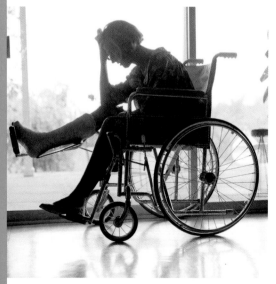

Is Stage Hypnosis Dangerous?

The key question that critics raise about stage hypnosis is whether it is potentially dangerous to members of the audience. The first concern is physical harm. There are anecdotal reports of participants bruising or even breaking limbs while performing some unusual action in a stage trance. These include the story of one man who was told by the stage hypnotist he was a ballet dancer and duly did the "splits," with very painful results.

In Britain a woman who was hypnotized during a stage show broke her leg after apparently jumping off the edge of the stage on her way to the bathroom. The young woman fell four feet, broke her leg in two places, and was in plaster for seven months. She later received about $30,000 in an out-of-court settlement.

In another case a young man who had eaten onions on stage after being told under hypnosis that they were apples became addicted to eating them; eating up to six raw onions a day. It took him several months to get over the habit.

More worrying, say the critics, is the second area of concern—that of potential psychological harm. They argue that stage hypnotists' concern is with entertainment, not to ensure that a hypnotized member of the audience can cope with the experience or has a chance to recover gently. This could be a problem if the subject shows some distress during the trance or if unwanted aspects of his or her life are brought out. This was the basis of a landmark court action in Britain in 2001 when a woman named Lynn Howarth successfully sued a stage hypnotist. Howarth, from Bolton in northwest England, had been one of a group of people hypnotized during a performance by the stage hypnotist Phil Damon (real name Philip Green). During the show she had regressed to her childhood and this had brought back memories of childhood abuse. Howarth claimed that the experience had left her depressed and a suicidal zombie and that she had twice tried to kill herself by driving her car at a tree. The judge awarded her compensation of the equivalent of around $10,000. The British government had already published guidelines in 1989 stating that stage hypnotists should not use age regression. Phil Damon claimed that he had followed the guidelines and that he had not used age regression. However, the judge ruled that the hypnotist's suggestion that Howarth imagine going back to being a child was negligent in the circumstances.

◗Anyone who volunteers to participate in stage hypnosis should have no fear of encountering physical or psychological damage.

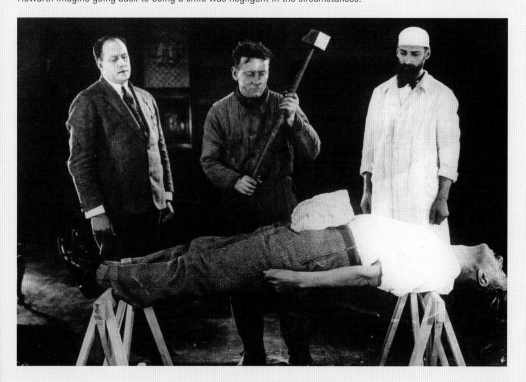

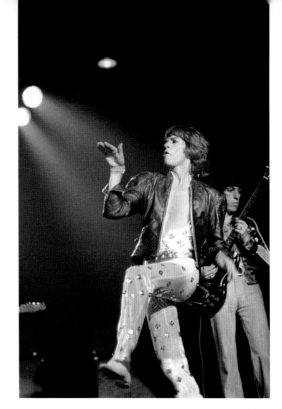

↶Getting a hypnotized member of the audience to sing and strut like a rock star, or quack like a duck, is all part of the show.

A high-profile court case which took place in 1998 involved the highly regarded British stage and television hypnotist Paul McKenna, who is also well known as a performer in the United States. McKenna had been sued by a furniture polisher, Christopher Gates, who claimed that his participation in one of McKenna's shows had induced schizophrenia. Gates had been admitted to the hospital nine days after featuring in the show at High Wycombe in central England, at which he had been convinced he could strut like the Rolling Stones singer Mick Jagger, talk in an alien language, and see through people's clothes using special glasses.

The judge rejected the claim, and said that it was "highly improbable" that Gates' illness had anything to do with his participation in the show. McKenna said the judgment was a vindication.

Probably the best-known case involving stage hypnosis and the law was that of Sharron Tabarn. Tabarn, aged 24, died five hours after being put in a trance at a show in a public house in Lancashire, northwest England, in 1993. The hypnotist had suggested to the woman that she would experience a 10,000-volt shock. Unknown to the hypnotist, Tabarn had a phobia of electricity. Five hours after the show she choked to death on her own vomit. Afterward, a local inquest into her death ruled that Tabarn had died from natural causes, and that she had probably had a seizure, which caused her choking. A court later ruled that, while they could not rule out the possibility that hypnosis had contributed to her death, there was insufficient reason to overturn the verdict of death by natural causes.

The tragedy did, however, lead to a review of the law on stage hypnosis by the British government and the formation of a new pressure group, set up by Tabarn's mother

Margaret Harper, called Campaign against Stage Hypnosis. Ultimately, however, a panel of experts set up by the government concluded that there was "no evidence of serious risk to participants in stage hypnosis, and that any risk which does exist is much less than that involved in many other activities."

A stage hypnotist named William Neal from Lehighton, Pennsylvania, was sued in 1997 after one of his shows. A female student, Nicole Henderson, said she was hit in the face by an unnamed male student after Neal, who performs under the name The Astonishing Neal, had put him in a trance. She alleged that, after Neal had told the male student to "do something to the person next to you that you would never think of doing," he turned around and punched Henderson in the face, cutting her below the left eye. She then filed a lawsuit in Luzerne County Court against Neal, seeking up to $40,000 in compensation. However, Neal's attorney, Anthony Roberti, gave a different explanation of what happened. He said, "They were leaving the stage and somehow his elbow got in the way of her face. It was an unavoidable incident." Roberti said Neal "had no control over that" and was in no way responsible for the accident.

The case was later settled out of court for an undisclosed sum with no admission of liability. Roberti said it was a "silly" case that should never have been brought. The debate continues about the effects of stage hypnosis, with some critics campaigning to have greater controls imposed or even to have stage hypnosis banned altogether.

Performers point out that there is nothing to fear from stage hypnotists who follow clear ethical guidelines about the safety and well-being of audience volunteers. Performers are taught to treat their subjects with respect and to ensure that any posthypnotic suggestions made during a show are removed when it ends.

Respect for the audience is the priority of stage performers. Their well-being and safety is paramount.

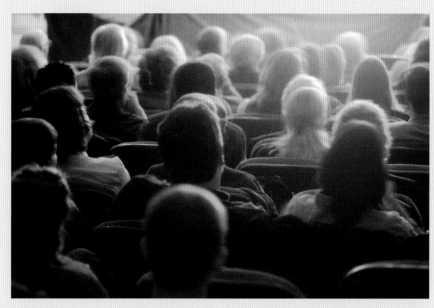

Stage hypnotists then and now

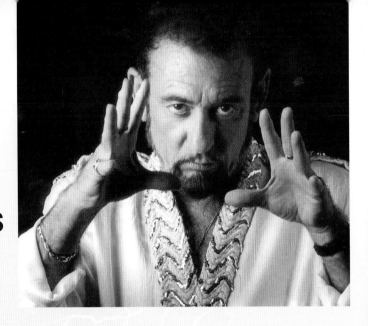

↳Martin St. James (pictured) is one of the great stars of twentieth-century stage hypnosis.

Figures of the Past

According to one of the grand figures of American hypnosis, Ormond McGill, it was stage hypnosis that helped maintain hypnosis in the public gaze at the end of the nineteenth century. At that time hypnosis was largely disregarded by the scientific establishment, as Freud's theories of psychoanalysis swept the world of psychology. It was only thanks to the work of the numerous showmen who flourished at the time, the theory goes, that hypnosis avoided disappearing into complete obscurity.

Since the time of Mesmer and mesmerism in the late eighteenth century, showmanship has gone hand in hand with the serious scientific study of hypnosis. Practitioners would often take part in elaborate stage shows and lectures in order to attract fee-paying patients. Hypnosis became a popular parlor game as the craze of mesmerism swept through Western countries. If the boundaries between the serious application of hypnosis and show business were sometimes blurred, so too were the lines between genuine hypnotists and charlatans who conned audiences into believing they were using the technique.

One figure who combined showmanship with healing and research was the Frenchman Charles de Lafontaine, a failed actor who discovered he had a gift for stage hypnosis—or mesmerism, as it was still usually called at the time. During his shows he was often accompanied on stage by a young boy, whom he would hypnotize. He would then demonstrate the boy's analgesia—inability to feel pain. On one occasion in the 1840s a skeptical member of the audience stabbed a scalpel into the boy's thigh to prove that the whole thing was a fraud, only to be astonished when the boy remained apparently unmoved.

Interestingly, it was the showmanship of de Lafontaine that helped inspire one of the most important early pioneers of hypnosis—James Braid. The Scottish physician went to one of the Frenchman's shows convinced that he was not going to be impressed, but instead became curious about the technique. Braid later became the first person to coin the phrase "hypnosis."

In the United States, the 1830s and 1840s saw a huge interest in mesmerism, which soon became adapted for stage shows. One offshoot was called "electrobiology," in which subjects would hold and stare at a small metallic disc in their hand, the idea being that electricity from the disc would mesmerize them. Among the American showmen who used this technique was one Dr. Darling. According to a contemporary report by an Englishman, Darling could make subjects experience cold items as hot, taste water as milk or brandy, see objects that were not there, forget their own names, and imagine themselves to be another person such as the Duke of Wellington or Prince Albert. All these phenomena are familiar ingredients of the modern stage-hypnotic repertoire.

Not all early stage hypnosis was so harmless. In a case reported in 1894, a European hypnotist, Franz Neukomm, took charge of a young woman named Ella Salamon, whom he had helped to heal of a nervous condition. Neukomm, who, like many hypnotists, combined showmanship with therapy, used Ella as his medium during a show. Typically, a member of the audience who was not well would come up on stage while Neukomm hypnotized the girl to empathize with the stage guest and find out from inside her mind what

Dr. Flint

Herbert L. Flint—or Dr. Flint as he styled himself—was one of the great pioneers of modern American stage hypnosis, developing a hugely popular touring show in the last decade of the nineteenth century. By today's standards, some of the routine was quite scary. Flint would suggest that a subject was being pursued by an angry swarm of bees, or had been struck by lightning, or even that the person had gone to hell. Other parts of the routine, such as making a male member of the audience fall in love with his "girlfriend"—really a broom covered with a cloth—are familiar today. According to some reports, a tragic accident occurred during one of Flint's shows, while he was on tour in Switzerland in the 1890s. In this particular routine, Flint would hypnotize his female assistant into a completely rigid state, place a rock on her laid-out body, and get a member of the audience to smash the rock with a hammer. On this occasion the member of the audience, perhaps from tension or overeagerness, missed the rock and hit the helpless woman's body. She later died from internal injuries. One report states that the poor woman on this occasion was none other than Flint's own wife.

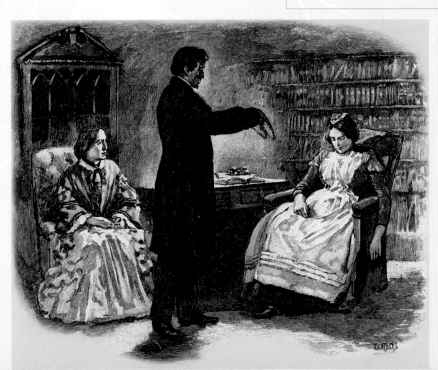

⌐Traditionally many of the "volunteers" in stage hypnosis were women, who were considered to be better hypnotic subjects than men.

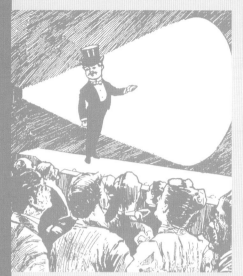

was wrong with her. This technique, known as channeling, was very common at the time. One night Neukomm slightly altered his suggestion to Ella and told her soul to leave her own body so that it could enter the patient's body. Twice, and unexpectedly, the hypnotized Ella resisted this new suggestion. Then Neukomm, frustrated by her refusal, deepened the girl's trance and commanded her soul once more to leave her body. Ella died during the session, and a postmortem examination suggested that she had died from heart failure probably caused by the hypnotic suggestion. Neukomm was duly charged with manslaughter and was subsequently convicted.

The great boom in stage hypnosis in the United States began in the 1890s with showmen such as Herbert "Dr." Flint, though even his shows were not without their tragedies (see page 113). The dominant figure in stage hypnosis for much of the twentieth century was Ormond McGill, known as the Dean of American Hypnotists, who was born in Palo Alto in 1913. As with many showmen of his time, he had first become interested in stage

∿Showmanship has gone hand in hand with the serious study of hypnosis since the late eighteenth century.

magic before concentrating on hypnosis. The author of numerous books, including the highly regarded *The New Encyclopedia of Stage Hypnosis,* McGill combined showmanship, scholarship, and therapy in his long career. He was also one of the first stage hypnotists to make use of the new medium of television and his work has inspired many of today's crop of stage performers all around the world. Other great stars of the twentieth century include Jimmy Grippo, the female performer Pat Collins, and the internationally known Martin St. James.

Today's Performers

There are now thousands of professional stage hypnotists working all over the world, with the most successful also appearing on television either as guests or on their own shows. For example, Jim Wand, a leading American hypnotist and comedian (with a Ph.D. in psychology) has appeared on "The Tonight Show with Jay Leno" and "The Late Show with David Letterman." The range of venues at which hypnotic entertainers perform is huge. Hypnotists can be found practicing their skill at fairs, graduations, banquets, conference events, private parties, and on cruise ships as well as at big entertainment venues such as Las Vegas.

The performances vary in their style and content, though humor is a central theme of most acts. Stage hypnotists always claim that the real stars of the shows are the volunteers, and it is this audience participation that gives such shows their unique, interactive atmosphere. Critics complain that some volunteers can suffer embarrassment or humiliation. In practice, however, most experienced performers go out of their way to avoid unnecessary embarrassment to clients, and audiences will be warned in advance what to expect. In some of the raunchier adult shows, for example, the audience will be informed that a certain amount of sexual byplay may be involved.

There are probably as many different stage-hypnosis routines as there are performers. Individual entertainers will have either their own unique set of suggestions, or at least their own variations of well-known ones. The basic pattern of each show might be quite similar: the volunteers are called up, put into a trance, and then a variety of suggestions and posthypnotic suggestions are put to their unconscious minds. The only limitation on the variety of the suggestions, however, is the imagination of the performer. Routines may include telling subjects that they are famous persons, telling them to talk like aliens, telling them to dance like Britney Spears or Tom Jones, telling them to use their shoes as telephones, telling them to see with the tips of their fingers, telling them to simulate an orgasm—the list goes on and on.

Terry Stokes

A good example of a current popular stage hypnotist is Terry Stokes. Since 1985 *The Terry Stokes Show* has toured the United States and Canada, playing a variety of venues, including the showrooms of Las Vegas. His act varies each time according to what happens on stage, but can include routines such as a man singing as if he were Dolly Parton or other volunteers taking part in a "car race" in their chairs. Stokes is a showman who enjoys being in front of an audience, using a blend of humor, charisma, and mystery to keep them entertained. Like many entertainers he started his career by studying hypnotherapy, but Stokes's strongest inspiration was watching the late American stage hypnotist Jack Berry perform in Atlanta in 1969. As with many top stage entertainers, Stokes has since added a title to his name, in his case, "America's Favorite Hypnotist."

Lady Hyp

Though stage hypnosis is still largely a masculine world, more and more women performers are starting to emerge. One of these is Christine Michele, the self-styled Lady Hypnotist—or Lady Hyp—from San Diego, who works out of Las Vegas. Her specialties include getting people to talk like Martians and making male volunteers think they are gorgeous supermodels. As is quite common among stage performers, Michele's original training was as a clinical hypnotherapist. Two great pioneers of female stage hypnosis were Joan Brandon, thought to be the first woman stage hypnotist, who reached the peak of her fame in the 1950s, and Pat Collins, a talented and glamorous entertainer who began performing in the 1960s and who became interested in the subject after she was cured of hysterical paralysis through the use of hypnosis.

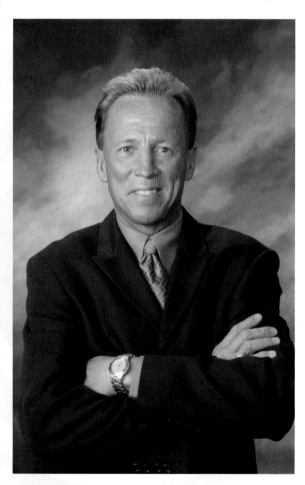

⤷Jim Wand (pictured) is a good example of the new breed of hypnotic performers who are equally at home on stage or on television.

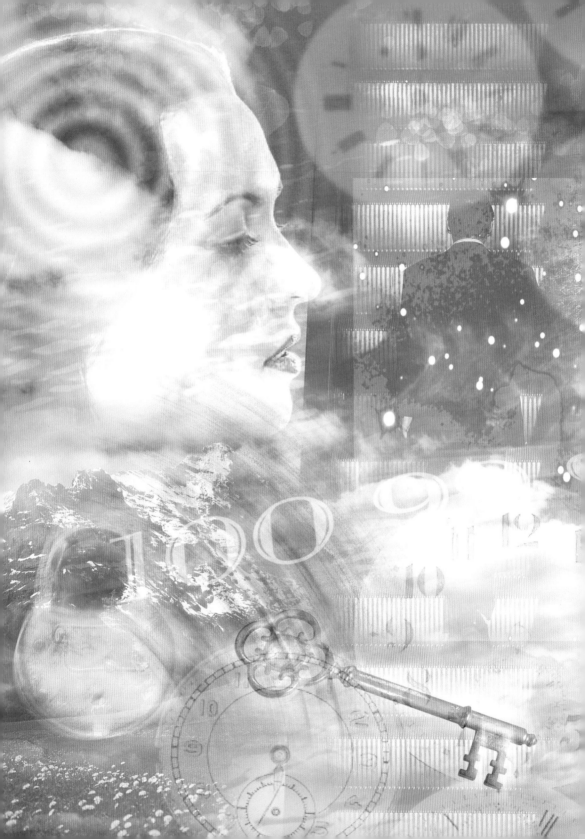

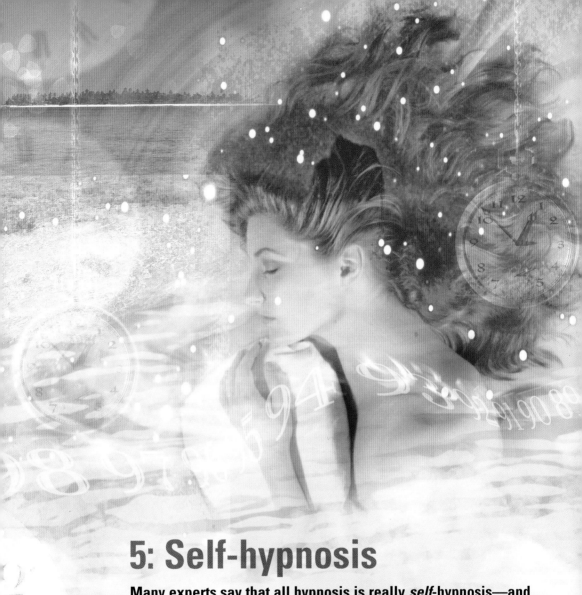

5: Self-hypnosis

Many experts say that all hypnosis is really *self*-hypnosis—and that you do not really need someone else to put you into a trance. The essential aspects of hypnosis—putting yourself into a trance, the use of suggestion—can be learned and applied in a straightforward manner. You may record the powerful induction and suggestion techniques yourself on tape or CD, or get a hypnotist or even a friend to do it instead. Here, look at how to unlock the potential of your unconscious mind, simply and safely, and discover for yourself the hidden power of hypnosis.

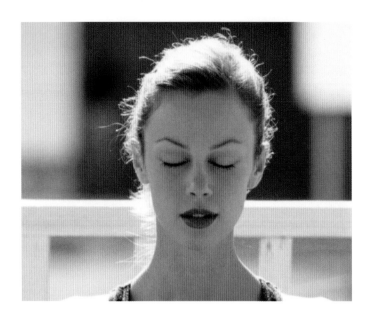

What is self-hypnosis?

Self-hypnosis, sometimes known as autohypnosis, is becoming increasingly popular and is used by many people to help them cope with the stresses of modern life.

So far, this book has dealt with hypnosis in which a person induces a trance in another person. This typical therapist-patient hypnosis is known as heterohypnosis. The subject for this section is self-hypnosis, or autohypnosis, which, as the name suggests, is the process whereby someone puts him- or herself into a trance. The obvious question is how does self-hypnosis differ from heterohypnosis? In many senses, there is no difference at all. Many expert hypnotists believe that all hypnosis is really self-hypnosis anyway. What they mean by that is that, while another person—the hypnotist—may be guiding you into a trance, it is your consciousness that is changing, not the hypnotist's. It is you, not the hypnotist, who is entering the trance. All the essential ingredients of hypnosis are present with the self-induced form, even if the means by which it is achieved are slightly different. These elements include the induction process, entering the trance, the suggestions for change, and leaving the trance.

There are some differences between the two forms of hypnosis. One of the most important is that in self-hypnosis there is no one there to make the suggestions to your unconscious mind during a hypnotic trance. In heterohypnosis this task is obviously performed by the hypnotist, using a prearranged script to meet the patient's particular needs. As will be discussed shortly, other strategies have to be adopted in self-hypnosis to deliver the suggestions in an effective way.

In the same way, people using self-hypnosis have no one else to put them into a trance. They have to do this themselves. This is the first main hurdle they

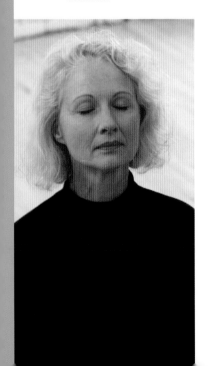

must overcome, and it is harder if they have never experienced a trance before in heterohypnosis. But putting yourself into a trance is by no means as difficult as it may sound.

Both these differences could be described as disadvantages of self-hypnosis, though they can be overcome simply enough. One distinct advantage may be in motivation. For any hypnosis to be successful, it helps if the person being hypnotized both believes that it will help and really wants it to help. This may not always be the case with people who are referred to a hypnotist by a practitioner or who have been persuaded to make an appointment by persistent friends or relatives.

With self-hypnosis, there may well be fewer doubts and higher motivation, for few people are likely to start self-hypnosis unless they really want it to work and believe it might.

Why Use Self-Hypnosis?

So why would anyone choose self-hypnosis? There may be several good practical reasons. Often a hypnotist will teach the client self-hypnosis as a way of reinforcing the initial treatment. Hypnosis is not a magical cure, and the effects can wear off if the beneficial suggestions are not reinforced on a regular basis. Therefore, learning how to put yourself into a trance can be a good way of ensuring that your initial treatment stays effective. This leads to the matter of cost. The fees vary, but trips to clinical hypnotists or hypnotherapists do not come cheap. The use of self-hypnosis can be a very cost-effective supplement or alternative to sessions with a therapist. There is also the question of availability— if you live in a remote area, there simply may be no qualified hypnotists near you. The choice then is either a long and expensive trip, or using the technique of self-hypnosis.

Another reason for mastering hypnosis is that your hypnotist cannot always be on hand when you need him or her most. If, for example, you have been visiting a therapist to help you control stressful situations, you cannot expect him or her to be there the next time your boss shouts at you or your truck breaks down on the highway. If the therapist has taught you self-hypnosis, however, or you have learned it, you can take charge of the situation yourself.

In any case, using self-hypnosis is a natural extension of the hypnosis process. Hypnosis can help you achieve your full potential—and what better way of doing this than by using the technique yourself?

Autogenic Training

Autogenic training (AT) is a fascinating offshoot of self-hypnosis. It was invented by a German scientist, Johannes Schultz (1884–1970), and uses relaxation and passive concentration to help improve a person's health. The idea is that the relaxation makes the central nervous system passive, allowing the autonomic nervous system to continue its control of the body's organs without distraction. During AT, the person focuses on the part of the body that needs treatment and repeats an appropriate phrase. In all, Schultz described six different verbal formulae, dealing with the arms, legs, head, abdomen, heart, and breathing. Regular practice is one of the keys to this technique, whose success has been demonstrated in medical studies. AT is popular in Germany and some other parts of Europe and its influence is growing. It has been shown to be effective in dealing with hypertension, anxiety, insomnia, circulation problems, and a range of other disorders.

⌣Autogenic training allows the autonomic nervous system to continue its control of the body's organs without interference from the central nervous system.

Is Self-Hypnosis Effective?

Two scientific studies have suggested that self-hypnosis may be just as effective as heterohypnosis. This proof is by no means conclusive, but the results, if correct, would not be surprising. If the quality and style of the suggestions are good enough, then there is no theoretical reason why a self-induced trance should not lead to good results, as good in some areas as a therapist-induced trance. In practice, of course, newcomers to self-hypnosis will need to take time to understand what they are doing, why they are doing it, and how best to achieve it.

What Are the Key Requirements?

To succeed with self-hypnosis, you do need to be motivated. If all you intend to do is lie down on a bed, switch on a tape, and wait for hypnosis to work its magic, then you may have a long wait in store. You cannot expect to get it right immediately and will need to practice often to perfect your technique. You should also want the hypnosis to work, and have at the least an open mind about whether it will, although the more you believe it will work, the faster it is likely to do so. Another requirement, and one that is hard for the modern skeptical mind to grasp, is to be as uncritical and accepting of the hypnosis technique as you can. Ideally, you want to stop consciously thinking or worrying about it, and just assume it will work. This mental approach will help open up your unconscious mind to suggestion, the key to success in hypnosis.

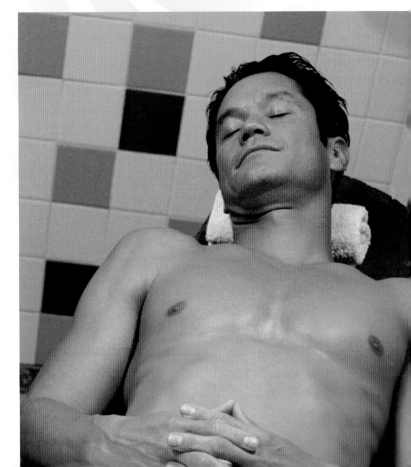

⤴Self-hypnosis is a technique that can easily be fitted into our busy lives, though it is easier to perform for the beginner if we can first find a quiet corner in which to relax.

Is It Easy?

The techniques of self-hypnosis are quite simple, but they are not easy. That is to say, there are no great mysteries in the methods and just about anyone can use them. However, as with all good things in life, self-hypnosis requires a certain amount of effort and application. You do need to practice, ideally every day and certainly very often. Gradually you will get used to feeling yourself go into a trance, and the more you become accustomed to this, the better you will be at inducing a trance and making it work for you.

Is Self-Hypnosis Dangerous?

Self-hypnosis is no more dangerous than heterohypnosis, which means to say it is not very dangerous at all, far less than just about any medication. However, one has to be careful in some circumstances. You should never use hypnosis tapes or CDs while you are operating machinery or driving a car or doing any activity that requires the full attention of the conscious mind. As with other types of hypnosis, anyone who has suffered mental illness should not use self-hypnosis unless this has the approval of a medical practitioner. Many hypnotists also advise against using self-hypnosis for age regression. This could bring up unwanted memories from the past without your having anyone qualified present to know how to handle the situation and reassure you. It is also not a good idea to use self-hypnosis to relieve pain until it is known what is causing that pain and you have, if appropriate, sought medical advice. For example, if you fracture your wrist but reduce the pain through hypnosis and continue to use that arm, you could risk causing yourself irreparable damage.

What about Self-Hypnosis Tapes and CDs?

The use of audiocassette tapes and CDs is of great benefit to anyone wanting to perform self-hypnosis because of the obvious difficulty in making suggestions to your unconscious mind while you are in a trance. Tapes and CDs can be made by the individual, or recorded by a therapist for general or a specific person's use, or even recorded by a friend using a script written by the individual concerned. There are literally thousands of prerecorded self-hypnosis tapes on the market, available via the Internet or mail order, covering a vast and diverse range of subject areas. However, the effectiveness of these recordings depends on their quality, and they are useful only as far as they address the particular needs of a person. This is why tailor-made recordings, ideally by a therapist or you under expert guidance, are best because they take into account not only your personality and the precise requirements you have, but also the results you are expecting from the self-hypnosis session.

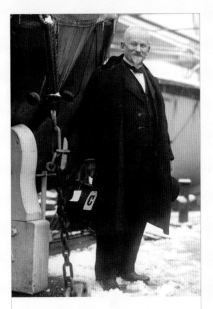

Autosuggestion

The Frenchman Émile Coué (pictured above, 1857–1926) who was an important student and early theoretician of hypnosis, popularized the idea of autosuggestion. His theory was that every person was the slave of suggestion, but could be freed by using a concept he described as "autosuggestion." This means replacing the negative suggestions that our minds have been subjected to during the course of our lives with positive suggestions that we ourselves propose. These affirmations, Coué believed, could transform our lives. He said that everything began in the mind, and that ideas we plant in the mind become real. His most famous affirmation was the one still widely familiar: "Day by day, in every way, I am getting better and better." Coué moved away from an emphasis on hypnosis to concentrate on autosuggestion; the latter is essentially a form of self-hypnosis without the trance.

Getting started

Before you attempt self-hypnosis, it is worth making a few preparations to boost your chances of success. The first thing to do is make sure you have some privacy and will be undisturbed while you put yourself into a trance. Once you are experienced, you will be able to perform self-hypnosis unaffected by the noise and distractions around you, but to start with make sure that cell phones, beepers, and other possible sources of interruption are switched off. If other people are in the house with you, make sure they understand your need to be undisturbed. If you are using tapes or CDs, try to listen through headphones, because they will cut back on other noises.

The next consideration is to make sure you perform the technique in a relaxed position. You might want to sit in an upright chair—it is best not to slouch—or lie down on your bed or couch or even on the floor. Make sure you are as comfortable as possible. If need be, use cushions and pillows to help you sit or lie still for up to half an hour. Also, make sure you go to the bathroom before you start so you will not be disturbed by a call of nature.

Another good tip is to perform a few stretching exercises for the muscles in your back, neck, arms, and legs before you start. These exercises are not essential, but will help to relax your body and prevent you from developing cramps in your muscles while you are undergoing the self-hypnosis.

It doesn't matter what you wear, or even whether you wear anything at all, but do make sure that any clothes are loose-fitting. You may want to remove your necktie or belt if they make you feel uncomfortable when you are lying

ϛSo that our bodies feel relaxed when we are sitting or lying down, it is a good idea to perform a few stretching exercises before we begin the self-hypnosis process.

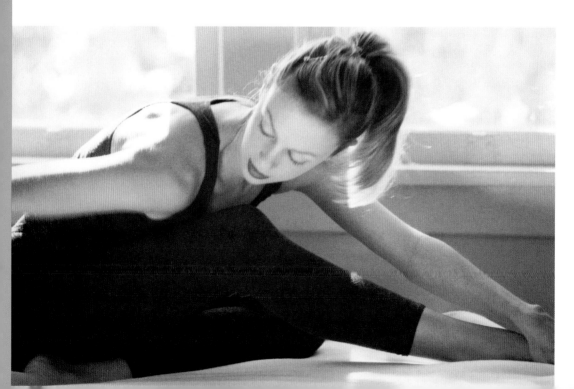

down or sitting upright. If you wear glasses, remove them, and if you use contact lenses it is advisable to take them out in case you should fall asleep after the session.

In the Dark

It is also a good idea to block out any strong sources of light. If you can, pull the curtains or blinds and turn off any very bright lights. Once you are more accomplished this will not be necessary, but it is good to give yourself the best possible start to your self-hypnosis routines.

One piece of equipment you might want to use is a timer, to make sure that you work within a set period. This does not matter if you are performing self-hypnosis before going to sleep. Don't worry, you cannot and will not get stuck in a trance, but it is possible that you will fall into a light sleep at the end of the trance, and if you don't want this to happen, then a timer is a useful safeguard. For your own comfort, do not use a timer with a very loud ring or buzz, because this might come as a bit of a shock!

If you really want to get your first few sessions off to the best possible start, then one idea is to play some relaxation or mood music before you commence the hypnosis. Music is sometimes also used as an aid during hypnosis itself.

Finally, do not become fixated on rules. The guidelines set out here are simply suggestions based on experience to help you achieve your goal of self-hypnosis. Do not be afraid to relax or amend them if another way suits you better. The more you think for yourself and find out what is best for you, then the better the self-hypnosis will be.

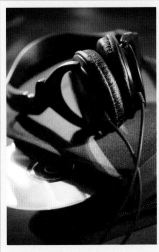

Using Music

Some people like to have music playing while they go into self-hypnosis because it can help the relaxation process and therefore the onset of trance. There is certainly nothing wrong with using music in this way, but be careful about what kind of music you choose. The music should be instrumental, not vocal—no human voices. It should also be rhythmic and relatively slow, not fast-paced or changing quickly in tempo. Do not play it too loudly and also be sure that the music does not have any bad associations for you, for example, reminding you of sad occasions or perhaps a broken relationship. Much Western or Indian classical music may be suitable, and there is also a wide variety of calming music available on the market. Recordings featuring the sound of waves gently breaking are particularly popular. Finally, make sure the tape does not end in the middle of your trance with a loud click.

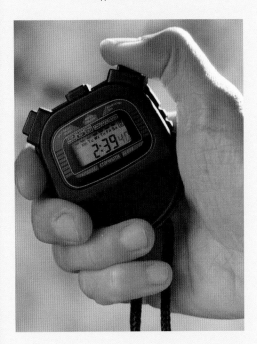

⌒If we are limited for time in our hypnosis sessions, a timer is a useful device to have, but try to avoid those with very loud bells or rings, as the shock of the noise may be discomforting.

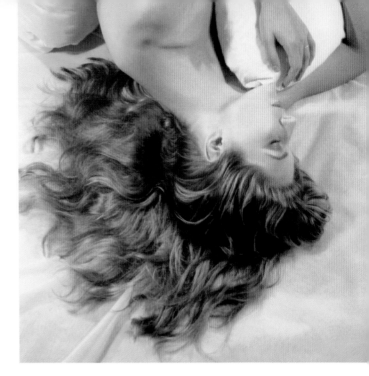

Getting into a trance

↪Hypnotic trance is not the same as falling asleep but it is important to make sure that you are in as comfortable a position as possible, whether this is sitting up or lying down.

You are now in a comfortable position, and ready to start your self-hypnosis program. How do you go into a trance? The process is called induction, and, as we discovered in an earlier section, there are numerous different techniques you can use. The essence of going into a trance is that you distract your conscious mind to allow your unconscious mind to come to the fore. The difference from heterohypnosis is that in self-hypnosis you have to do the distraction yourself. Since most hypnotists believe that all hypnosis is essentially self-hypnosis, there is no theoretical obstacle to this. In practice, it simply means that the induction techniques have to be altered a little.

One way of approaching induction is using audiocassettes or CDs. These might be recorded by you from a script that you have either written yourself or obtained and adapted from another source. Alternatively, you might want to use a tape from your hypnotist, if you have one, or from one of the many prerecorded tapes and CDs that are on the market. The advantage of this approach is that you are listening to an "outside" voice and do not have to worry about talking or visualizing yourself into a trance. The disadvantage is that you may find the speed of the tape induction too slow or too fast.

The other option is to do the induction yourself, in your mind, perhaps with the aid of a physical object on which to focus your attention. In this case, you will be able to control the speed at which you progress. In theory, there is a contradiction between "you" and the individual trying consciously to put "yourself" into a trance. In practice, however, doing the induction yourself, in your own mind, is possible because we can naturally dissociate one part of the mind from another.

Whether you are creating your own induction, getting a hypnotist to record it for you, or buying a ready-made tape, you will want to consider what form of words works best for you. The direct approach is where the words tell you or instruct you what to do and what you are feeling; for example, "You are now feeling relaxed, you can feel the relaxation in your legs." The indirect or permissive approach is more subtle. In the same example you might use the words, "You may notice how relaxed you are, and may be aware of relaxation in your legs." Neither approach is right or wrong, although some individuals respond better to one style rather than the other.

After performing an induction technique, you should feel very relaxed and your eyes will be closed. Technically, this is known as "neutral hypnosis," during which you are in a trance but without suggestions having yet been put to your unconscious.

Progressive Relaxation

One of the most common and easy-to-learn induction techniques, and a good one to start with, is progressive relaxation.

When you are comfortable and ready to start, begin to imagine your body as it slowly relaxes from one end to the other; you can start from either the head or the feet. Imagine the sensation that your feet are feeling very relaxed, as if a stream of relaxation were flowing through them. As you become aware of your feet relaxing, first one and then the other, tell yourself that you are moving into a trance. Notice how the stream of relaxation is gradually flowing through your body, relaxing one body part after another, taking you deeper into a trance. Continue this process until you have completed the whole of your body, not forgetting your arms and hands.

On page 139 there is an example of a progressive relaxation induction script that you could tape or ask someone else to tape for you. It would also be easy simply to talk yourself through the script in your head; you don't need to memorize all the words so long as you follow the general pattern of the instructions.

Other Techniques

The progressive-relaxation method is among the easiest and most reliable to use, but it is certainly worth trying out other techniques to see which suit you best. There are many methods to get you into a trance, and all of them work by shutting off sensations from the outside world and focusing your attention on you and your internal body sensations.

Speaking Your Name

One technique that may help you use taped recordings of inductions and suggestions more effectively is to make sure that you are addressed with your own name, instead of just as "you." So, for example, if your name is Susan you might say, "Susan, as you walk down the staircase, step by step, you are moving deeper and deeper into a trance." It may feel a little strange to record a script that is tailored so personally, or to listen to such a recording by someone else, but research has suggested that individuals do respond powerfully to the use of their own names.

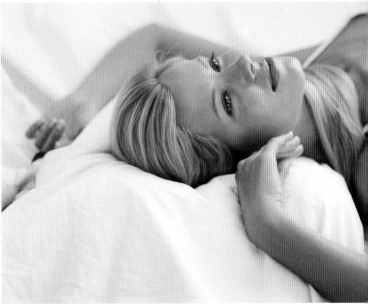

One straightforward way to induce a trance is to focus on your body as it becomes progressively and slowly relaxed.

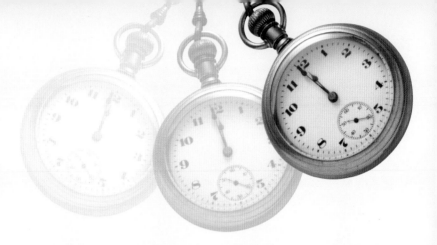

↪A watch has no magical properties when it comes to inducing hypnosis, but focusing on a particular object is a good way of going into a trance.

↪Another induction technique is to hold something in your hand such as a key or coin and then gradually feel your grip becoming looser and looser.

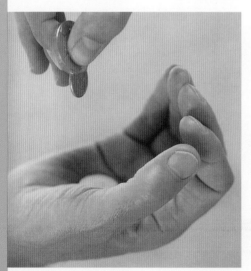

Staring at an Object

Concentrate on an object that is just above eye level, which you can see without straining your neck. Stare at the object and take slow, deep breaths.

Tell yourself that your body is feeling warm and relaxed. Notice how your arms and legs are starting to feel a little heavy. As you are breathing slowly, in and out, be aware how relaxed you are feeling, how the relaxation is spreading all over your body. Notice that as you keep staring, and staring at the object, you are feeling more and more relaxed. Tell yourself that as this warm feeling of relaxation grows, as you keep staring, you are moving deeper into a trance. Notice, too, how your eyelids are beginning to feel pleasantly relaxed and heavier, and that as you keep breathing, in and out, it is becoming harder and harder to keep them open. As you keep staring, the pleasant feeling of relaxation is spreading all over your body.

Continue staring and breathing in this way until finally your eyes close and you feel deeply relaxed and comfortable.

Holding an Object

In this technique you hold a small object—perhaps a coin—in your hand and stretch your arm out in front of you. Concentrate on your thumbnail, and keep staring at it. Then tell yourself you are becoming more and more relaxed, and that when your arm and your hand, and then your fingers, become relaxed, your fingers will open. Tell yourself again that as your fingers become more relaxed they will open and release the coin, and that the falling coin will be the sign that you are going deeply into a trance. Keep repeating these words, and feel your grip on the coin becoming looser and looser, until your fingers are so loose that they open and the coin is gently released. Once you have dropped the coin your eyes will be closed and you will be in a trance. Your arm will fall gently to your side, you will feel more and more relaxed, going deeper and deeper into a trance.

The Staircase

Another popular method is to imagine yourself at the top of a staircase. Close your eyes and watch yourself walking slowly, step by step, down the staircase. It can be any kind of staircase you like; just make sure it has no bad associations. Count each step as you walk slowly down, watching yourself all the time. Tell yourself that as you slowly go down, you will be feeling more and more relaxed, and moving deeper and deeper into a trance. Imagine that as you reach the bottom of the staircase, you will feel completely relaxed and be deep in the trance.

There are a number of variations of the staircase method, including starting at the bottom and walking up if that suits you better. If stairs are not your thing, then why not try a long tree-lined avenue that you walk along, counting the trees one by one as you pass them? Maybe the avenue will run up or down a slight hill, maybe it won't. You decide.

A Beautiful Place

Another technique is to imagine yourself in a beautiful place where you feel particularly comfortable. It might be a beach, a little wood, a meadow, in a favorite garden, or by a river. Now imagine yourself relaxing, as in previous exercises. You might want to count slowly to ten in your mind; with each number you will be aware of some new detail at the scene. Become engrossed in what is around you. Tell yourself you are relaxed, and that with each number, with each new detail, you are moving deeper and deeper into a trance.

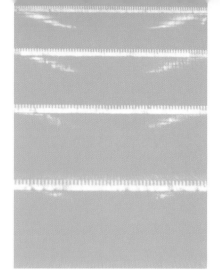

↶A popular way of inducing a trance is to imagine yourself slowly walking down—or up—a staircase.

Practicing the Skill

Self-hypnosis is a skill, and like any skill it needs to be learned and practiced. You cannot expect to master a skill in just one attempt, so try to set some time aside each day to practice. It need not be a long period—20 or even 10 minutes a day is enough to make good progress. It is best if you get into a routine and use the same time of day. This might be when you first get up, before you go to sleep, or when you get home from work. When you practice, however, beware of trying too hard. As with falling asleep, the trick of self-hypnosis is just to let your mind go, adopting the attitude that what will be, will be. Simply perform the induction technique, without worrying about what you want to achieve.

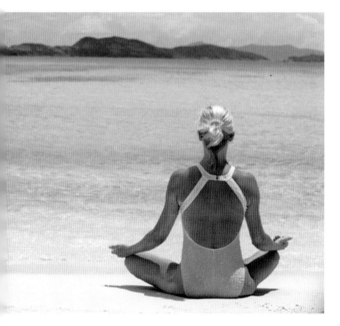

↶Perhaps one of the most pleasant ways to bring about or enhance a trance is by imagining yourself in a beautiful location, either real or imaginary.

Reawakening and deepening the trance

Once you are in a trance, the next step usually is to deepen it and then apply the suggestions to your unconscious mind. We will be considering both shortly. However, you may want to practice going in and out of the trance before you move on to the suggestions, so it is useful to consider reawakening first.

When you leave your trance you are not technically reawakening because you were not asleep in the first place. However, "awakening" and "reawakening" are commonly used expressions in hypnosis. Reawakening is a very simple process, and can be achieved in a number of ways. If you are using a timer, simply tell yourself that when the timer goes off you will start to come slowly and gently back to the waking or regular state and that when you have finished counting one to ten you will be awake, feeling relaxed. Another way, without the timer, is also to suggest that you will start counting slowly to ten (or whatever number you choose) and that as you start counting you will come gradually and peacefully out of the trance, and that when you reach ten you will awaken feeling totally refreshed.

If you have used a staircase or other similar induction technique, then you can imagine yourself walking back up (or down, as the case may be). You will tell yourself that as you walk back up you will slowly be coming out of the trance, until you reach the top, when you will awaken, refreshed.

Deepening the Trance

Once you have put yourself into a trance, the next step is to try to deepen it. There is nothing mysterious about this. Generally speaking, the deeper you get into a trance, the more success your suggestions will have. A good technique is to take advantage of the world around you. Though you will have done your best to find a quiet spot in which to perform self-hypnosis, it is very hard to exclude all noises. While in a trance you might hear aircraft, traffic noise, a neighbor's dog, or other sounds. These do not have to be a problem; in fact, you can make use of them to deepen your trance. Tell yourself that with each

Outside noises, such as aircraft or a passing automobile, can be a distraction during hypnosis; but by incorporating them into your trance you can actually turn them to your advantage.

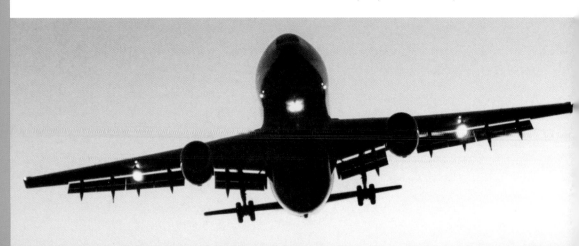

aircraft passing, or with each bark of the dog, you are going deeper into a trance. This can be a very powerful method of deepening. Much of what you want to achieve through self-hypnosis can be achieved in a relatively light trance; however, deepening the trance gives you a good feel for the trance state, as you come to know the difference between one stage of hypnosis and another. The more familiar you become with how you feel in the trance, the better you will be at self-hypnosis.

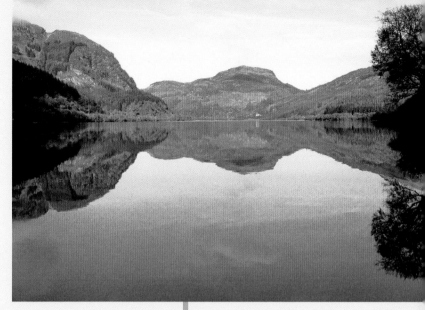

Deepening techniques work in much the same way as induction methods. The use of counting is a very familiar one, as you tell yourself that with each number you are going deeper into a trance. Or you may use the staircase example, and start ascending or descending another staircase. With each step you will tell yourself you are going deeper into your hypnotic state.

Do not worry about getting stuck in a trance. It cannot and will not happen. The worst that can happen is that you doze off for a few minutes. It is a good idea to tell yourself that you will feel alert and refreshed when you come out of the trance. Your unconscious will respond to this suggestion, and that is how you will feel.

How Do I Know I Was in a Trance?

Quite often people who try self-hypnosis for the first time wonder whether they were really in a trance. They will be perplexed that they were still conscious and their mind alert. Can this be hypnosis? The answer is yes. The main physical symptom of being in a trance is a deep sense of relaxation. Though your mind may be very still, it will still be aware. Hypnosis is not something weird or bizarre: it feels—and is—a perfectly natural state. You should monitor how you feel during the hypnosis and afterward; perhaps you can keep a written record. There is no one fixed feeling that all people have when they are hypnotized. People vary in their sensations, and the experience may change the deeper you are in a trance. As you practice self-hypnosis you'll learn to be aware of what you can expect to feel in different stages of hypnosis.

Using Visualization

Along with verbal commands, direct and indirect, visualization is a way of communicating with the unconscious mind. It is implicit in much of what people do when they induce or deepen a trance or make suggestions: they are picturing a scene. Visualization exercises are a good way of practicing your self-hypnosis skills. After inducing a trance you can take yourself into a favorite scene—it does not have to be real or somewhere that you have actually visited—and look around. Picture the scene in your mind's eye and notice the detail of your surroundings. As you do so, tell yourself you are going deeper and deeper into a trance. Stay in this imaginary world for some minutes. Then, when you are ready, you can slowly move away from the scene and reawaken yourself in the usual way.

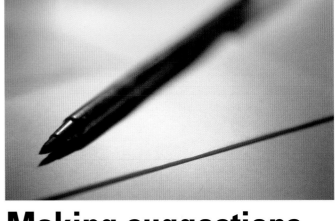

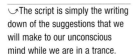
↳The script is simply the writing down of the suggestions that we will make to our unconscious mind while we are in a trance.

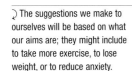
♪ The suggestions we make to ourselves will be based on what our aims are; they might include to take more exercise, to lose weight, or to reduce anxiety.

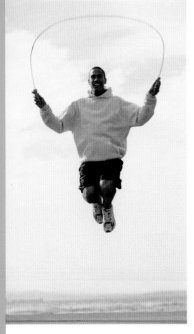

Making suggestions and writing scripts

You are in a comfortable position and have gone into a trance. What now? A trance state on its own—what is called neutral hypnosis—may induce a feeling of well-being and relaxation. But to achieve your goals you need actively to reprogram your unconscious mind. This can be done through the use of hypnotic suggestions.

Setting Your Goals

First of all, you have to work out what your aims are. What do you want to achieve from hypnosis? You might want to become better at speaking in public or more confident at social gatherings, perhaps reduce your tendency to worry, learn to be more tolerant, lose weight, give up smoking, take more exercise, or any one of many other aims. Write down what it is in your case. In general, it is better to be quite specific in your aims. Simply saying, "I want to be happy" is vague and very hard to quantify. Think about particular areas of your life you want to improve, or how you want to feel in response to certain situations. You need not worry, however, if your aim is understood only by you and might not make sense to someone else. If that is what you want, then your unconscious mind will understand what you mean.

Formulating a Suggestion

Once you have decided what your goal is, then you can begin to formulate the suggestion. A suggestion may be just one sentence or it may be several hundred words long. These longer suggestions are called "scripts" because for practical reasons they are usually written down. When you are trying self-hypnosis for the first time it is probably a good idea to start with the shorter, more straightforward suggestions before working your way to longer scripts, but this is up to you. It is harder to use longer scripts for self-hypnosis without the aid of CDs or tapes, though it is certainly possible.

As with deciding upon your goal, the key to effective suggestions is to be specific and where possible use as much detail as you can. Suppose, for example, that you have a problem with losing your temper when you are driving, blaming all other road users apart from yourself. So you want to stop losing control each time you sit behind the wheel. You could just use, "I want to control my temper" as your suggestion, but that is quite vague. You should try to be more specific.

Think again about your goal and write it down: "I want to be able to control my temper while driving my car." Then consider the kind of behavior that will help you toward your goal: "I will keep calm, peaceful, and in a serene but alert state of mind while I am driving." Next, think of a way to help you achieve this new kind of behavior: "When I get into my car I will put on some peaceful, relaxing music and this will keep me calm and serene."

If you put these words together you will come up with a short suggestion that will start to change your behavior while you drive. It may read, "I will keep my temper in my car if I stay in a calm, peaceful, serene but alert state of mind. So when I get into my car I will switch on some peaceful, relaxing music, and this will keep me calm."

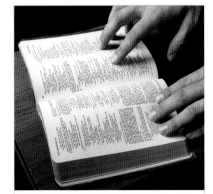

ⒸIt is all too easy to lose our temper while we are driving; but by using self-hypnosis we can learn to control our rage.

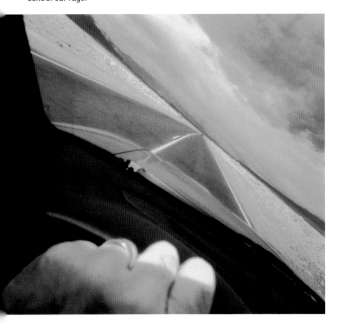

Alternative Suggestions

If you are someone who is interested in the sayings of great people and writers, then you could try using famous quotations as your suggestions during a trance. These act as indirect rather than direct suggestions and will engage the curiosity of your unconscious. If such quotations hold a deep meaning for you, and express some value or quality you would like to attain, then this can be a powerful technique, no matter how general the quotations seem to others. For example, if you want to build up your sense of individuality and gain the courage to make your own decisions, you could use a well-known quotation from one of William Shakespeare's plays:

"This above all: to thine own self be true,
And it must follow, as the night the day,
Thou canst not then be false to any man."
(*Hamlet*, Act 1, Scene 3.)

Alternatively, you may choose a quotation from Jesus. For example:

"What good is it for a man to gain the whole world, yet forfeit his soul?"
(Mark 8: 36, New International Version.)

Choose the quote that has most relevance to you.

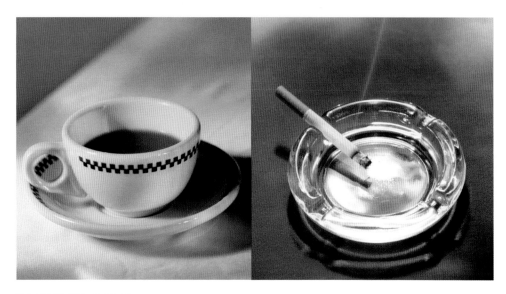

⌒Certain activities can act as triggers for our bad habits. For example, we may feel like having a cigarette every time we have a cup of coffee. The aim of the suggestion is to replace that bad response with another, healthier one— for example, to feel like eating an apple or drinking a glass of water.

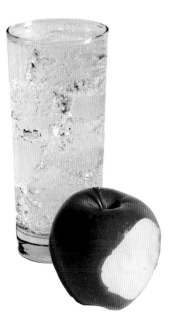

Setting the Trigger

The previous page is a very simple example of how to build up a simple suggestion. It has a specific aim and works toward that aim. Do not be afraid to use your own words to express yourself, as your own unconscious mind will understand what you want, in the context you want it. In fact, this is one way that self-hypnosis can be every bit as powerful as hypnosis by another person or using prerecorded tapes. You know, deep down, what you really want to achieve, and that knowledge will help you find the words to express it in the right way for you.

Notice that in this example of driving the act of turning on the music achieves two ends. The chances are that the soothing sounds will help relax you as you are driving. But more importantly, it will be the trigger for the suggestion that you will feel calm and relaxed when you do this. This is an example of a posthypnotic suggestion.

Some people get alarmed by the idea of posthypnotic suggestions, a fear prompted perhaps by too many Hollywood movies and some of the more lurid stage-hypnosis shows. In fact, many of the therapeutic suggestions used in hypnosis are posthypnotic.

For example, suppose you are a smoker and want to give it up. The trouble is, every time you have a cup of coffee you feel like having a cigarette with it. That is your trigger for smoking. So your hypnotic suggestion may be that in the future, when you have a cup of coffee you will no longer feel like having a cigarette but instead will want to eat an apple, drink a glass of water, or perform some other harmless activity. This is an example of a posthypnotic suggestion, in other words a suggestion that takes effect after the hypnosis and at the prompting of a trigger or signal, in this case drinking coffee. A different approach to smoking might be the suggestion that you no longer enjoy smoking and that each time you try to smoke a cigarette it makes you feel nauseated.

At the end of this chapter (see pages 139–141) there are some longer self-hypnosis scripts, which you can adapt for your own purposes.

Imagination and Visualization

Imagination plays a central role in hypnosis. If words are the language of the conscious mind, then imagination is the language of the unconscious mind. The unconscious responds powerfully to stories and images, so it is important to make as much use of the imagination as possible when working with suggestions. The ability to visualize during

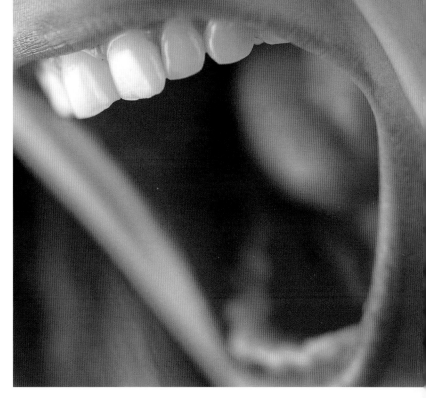

Instead of automatically responding with anger to stressful trigger situations such as driving, we can teach ourselves to react in a calm, relaxed manner.

133

hypnosis, and to see yourself behaving in the way you want to, is very effective. When you are in a trance, you can either do an unscripted take-it-as-it-comes visualization or script it in advance to help with the detail. This is where the inclusion of detail in scripts is very useful. You can describe scenes that will appeal to your imagination, making them as vivid as you can.

Let us take our previous example of bad temper and driving. Try to visualize yourself in the car, driving along, with the feel of the steering wheel in your hands, looking at the road signs, listening to the noises of the traffic. Then imagine the calmness you feel while the soothing music is playing. The more detail you can imagine, the more powerful the suggestions will be.

Your unconscious mind responds particularly well to symbolic or metaphorical stories. These stories will outwardly be about someone or something else, but inwardly describe a process that affects you. Your unconscious mind will understand the true meaning of these stories, after all, you will have chosen the story in the first place. For example, while you may be telling yourself a story about removing weeds from the garden, your unconscious mind will interpret this correctly as really being about getting rid of the parts of your life which make you unhappy. Think about a story that has affected you deeply and that has some relevance to what you are trying to achieve, perhaps a fairy tale like "Cinderella," or some other powerful tale. Adapt it into a script if it fits your needs, or perhaps try to make up a simple symbolic story yourself.

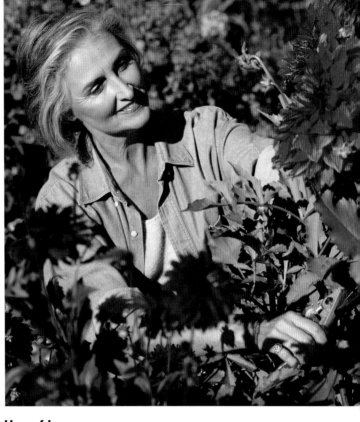

↪For many people, imagining they are in a peaceful location such as a garden can be a powerful tool in their self-hypnosis sessions.

Use of Language

When you are constructing the sentences of your script, try to avoid negative words and expressions. For example, it is better to say, "You will stop feeling less happy" than to say, "You will stop feeling sad." The unconscious mind picks up on words, and it is better for it to hear "happy" than "sad." It is best to use positive words wherever possible. You do not have to worry about being grammatical, because the unconscious mind will work out what you mean from the key concepts you are using. In fact, a little confusion is no bad thing, because this can help you bypass the conscious mind, which doesn't make sense of what you are saying, and reach the unconscious, which does. For example you might abruptly end a sentence in the middle, or add a random question such as, "Isn't that right?" for no apparent reason.

If you look at the scripts at the end of this chapter, you will see how the words used are measured and deliberate, with repetitions and pauses to punctuate the flow. The language is not quite grammatical, and this does not matter. The words are trying to bypass your conscious mind and instead appeal directly to your unconscious mind, with the prompting of key words.

Another technique used in writing scripts is to give the mind the illusion that you are offering choice; this helps to keep it focused on what you are suggesting. So you might say in a visualization exercise, "As you reach the beautiful garden, you may feel inner peace, or perhaps have a feeling of great tranquility." There really isn't a difference in the choices, but the mind believes it has a choice to make.

Consider also whether you are likely to respond better to direct or indirect suggestions. The "commands" you make do not have to be direct: they can be "embedded." For example, you might say, "You are feeling calm," which is direct. Or you could say, "People who reach this point usually notice they are feeling calm." The command to feel calm is still there, but embedded. When spoken, the words can be emphasized slightly, making them stand out for your unconscious. Often, the unconscious mind seems to respond better to these more subtle command triggers than to direct, head-on instructions.

Delivering the Script

If you want to use quite a long script, it may be better if you record it (or someone else records it for you) onto an audiocassette or CD, and then play this to yourself under hypnosis. You can also record an induction sequence, and do not forget to add your reawakening at the end.

The reason why a recording might be better is that it avoids your having to read from a script while you are in trance. While this is possible, it is probably easier for you to start by using a tape. The other option is for you to remember the script and say it to yourself while you are in hypnosis. Again, this is possible, and you do not have to worry about getting it right word for word; it is the meaning that counts.

Key Points for Suggestions

- Use simple language and be specific

- Be as imaginative as you can and as vivid in detail as possible

- Repetition of key words and phrases can be very powerful

- Leave pauses for the words to sink in and deepen your trance

- Your unconscious mind will understand what you mean

- Try to avoid negative words and phrases

- Metaphors and stories are a good way of talking to your unconscious mind

- Make your own recordings for long scripts

135

◝Modern technology is a great help to mastering self-hypnosis, as we can use audiocassettes or CDs to record our scripts and then play them back to ourselves.

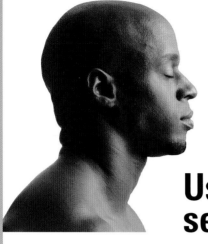

Uses of self-hypnosis

⤸There are potentially limitless uses of self-hypnosis once we have learned to focus on the power of the unconscious mind.

↧ One of the most common uses of self-hypnosis is to help quit smoking; many smokers have found the technique very effective.

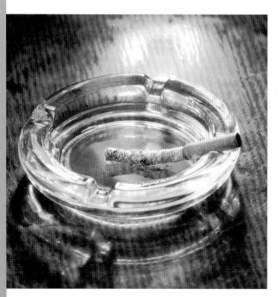

Self-hypnosis can be a valuable tool in helping change your life for the better. One of the principal advantages is that, because you are doing it yourself, you are simply able to use self-hypnosis much more often than if you were visiting a hypnotist. This frequency is important. Hypnosis is not an instant wonder cure. It is unrealistic to expect to change habits that have built up over 10, 20, or 30 years in one short session of self-hypnosis. Frequent sessions, however, can produce real and lasting change. It is true that some very experienced hypnotists can change a patient's behavior in just one session. A number, indeed, offer one-time sessions lasting 90 minutes or less in which they claim to be able to stop a person from smoking, and this can work. Quite often, however, an ingrained habit such as smoking may require three or four separate sessions to conquer it.

The specific uses of self-hypnosis are many and varied, but here are a few of the most common ones. You can try out different areas yourself, but please make sure you stick to the following guidelines: If you are suffering any kind of medical condition that might require expert attention, do seek that medical advice before you even consider hypnosis. The same also applies if you are suffering, or have suffered, any serious psychological disorders.

Stopping Smoking

Hypnosis has been shown to be very effective in helping individuals quit smoking. The suggestions you make can be to replace your urge to smoke with other, less harmful, activities. You might, for instance, suggest that when you feel the urge to smoke you will instead drink water or go for a walk.

Additionally, you could remind your unconscious of the real benefits of being an ex-smoker: you will live longer, feel healthier, taste food better, and save money. Another approach is aversion: suggest that when you try to smoke a cigarette it will make you feel nauseated. Choose the approach that suits you. (See page 140 for a sample script to help you stop smoking.)

Also, give yourself a better chance by taking some other practical steps. When you are in the process of giving up, try for a while to avoid situations where you might be especially tempted to smoke. Don't leave cigarettes lying around, and involve your family and friends in your efforts. It is also good to make the suggestion to your unconscious mind that if you are in the company of someone smoking you will be tolerant, but will not feel tempted to smoke a cigarette yourself.

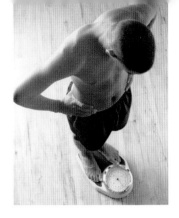

⤵If you are struggling to lose weight why not try self-hypnosis?

Losing Weight

The two ways to lose weight are to consume less of the wrong kinds of food and drink and to take more exercise. Self-hypnosis can help you achieve both—and with lasting effect. Use the power of suggestion to increase your resolve to eat less junk food, to eat healthier food such as fresh fruit, vegetables, and complex carbohydrates, and to stop snacking on foods when you are watching television, or at a movie. Tell yourself that you will stop eating when you are full, that you will drink lots of water, and that you will eat regularly and not late at night.

Generally, people do not have a problem losing weight, but they do when it comes to keeping it off. You can use hypnosis to add resolve to your diets. Make the suggestion that when you start to feel a craving for junk food you will do some exercise instead, and use visualization to "think thin." If you are very overweight, make sure you consult your medical practitioner before taking strenuous exercise.

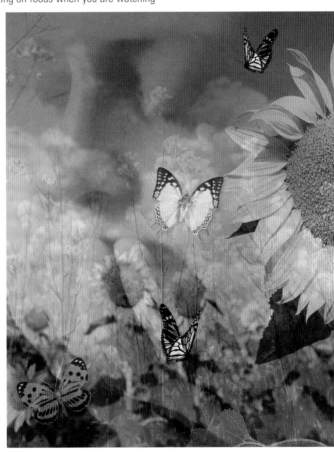

⤶Visualizing yourself in a beautiful, tranquil place will help you get to sleep at night.

Sleeping Better

The inability to get to sleep—insomnia—can be very distressing. Self-hypnosis can be very effective in overcoming this problem. During a trance, try simple suggestions, telling yourself that you will have a good night's sleep, that you will sleep peacefully and normally through all normal noises, and, unless you have to wake before, you will awaken in the morning feeling alert and refreshed. Or you could use a visualization technique just before you want to go to sleep, imagining yourself in a beautiful place, feeling deeply relaxed and calm, and observing your enchanting surroundings. (See page 141 for a sample script to help you sleep better.)

Building Self-Confidence

Self-hypnosis is effective in building self-confidence and reducing general anxiety. You might use short suggestions, perhaps the famous quotation from the French pioneer of autosuggestion Emile Coué: "Day by day, in every way, I am getting better and better." Or make up some short ones of your own, telling yourself that you are growing in confidence, that as each day passes you are coping with problems better, feel less nervous and more in command.

Alternatively, you might want to use a longer script, perhaps based on visualization and words, imagining yourself confident, strong, and worry-free in all situations. Remember, you are the person who really knows what you want and what you need, so you are ideally suited to coming up with the right suggestions yourself.

Improving Memory

You can use self-hypnosis to improve your memory, help you study better, take tests with confidence, speed-read, and master new skills. Before you study, suggest to yourself during a trance that you will work efficiently, that you will remember and understand what you study. You might say that when you start reading a study book you will read more quickly than usual, concentrating more and understanding and recalling more.

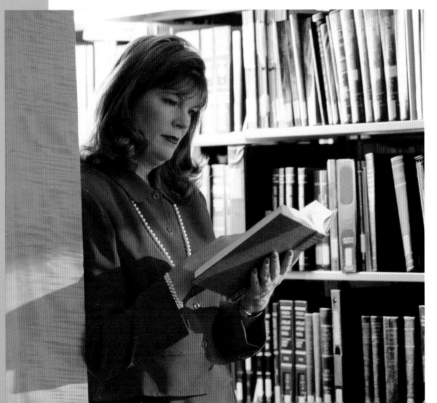

Before important tests you can use the suggestion that, at the time you sit down in front of the paper, you will be able to remember in detail what you have studied, and you will feel relaxed and able to deal calmly with any question that you encounter. Self-hypnosis may not turn you into a Nobel-prizewinning scholar, but it can and will help you realize your true potential. (See page 141 for a sample script to help you perform better on tests.)

⟨ If you have trouble concentrating when studying, self-hypnosis could be the solution.

Sample scripts

Hypnosis scripts vary in length and style and you will come to understand which work best for you. Here are some examples of different scripts that you can learn from and adapt for your own needs. We start with an induction, then move on to scripts for suggestions. When you record or read a script, or repeat it in your head, remember to say the words in a slow, measured voice with a steady tone. Use plenty of pauses (they are marked with three dots in the script below) and don't be afraid to repeat phrases.

1. Induction

This is the progressive-relaxation method. If you record it, or get someone else to record it, change "I" to "you." If you simply repeat the script in your head, you don't have to memorize every word so long as you recreate the pattern of the instructions. Speak in a slow voice, and leave pauses where indicated. Some people prefer not to use the word "trance" but prefer to say "sleep," even though hypnosis is not the same as sleep. In that case it's a good idea to use phrases such as "special sleep" or "hypnotic sleep." Don't worry, your unconscious will know what you mean.

I have the sensation of my feet, feeling very relaxed. It is as if a stream of relaxation is flowing through my feet. A stream of relaxation is flowing through my feet. Gradually flowing to the rest of my body. As I am aware of my feet becoming, relaxed, so I am moving gradually, gently, safely, into a trance … Now my feet are very relaxed, and that relaxation is flowing into my legs. And I can feel how relaxed my feet are becoming. First my right foot, slowly becoming relaxed. Then my left foot, becoming slowly relaxed. As I breathe slowly in. And out. Breathe in, and breathe out. I notice how this relaxation is flowing, gradually, up my legs. I am aware that as my legs become more, and more, relaxed, so I am gradually moving deeper, deeper, safely, into a trance … Now I can feel

that relaxation flowing, from my feet, from my legs, into my pelvis. I feel my pelvis becoming relaxed. As the stream of relaxation spreads through my legs, into my pelvis, I am gradually moving deeper, deeper, into a trance. Now, the relaxation is flowing through my legs and pelvis. As I breathe in, breathe out, slowly. Breathing in, out, slowly … And as I breathe in, out, slowly, I am aware that I am falling gently, safely, into a trance. Now, I feel that stream of relaxation flowing from my legs, my pelvis, and into my abdomen. I feel that stream of relaxation, flowing smoothly, gently, into my abdomen. As the relaxation flows into my abdomen I am aware how I am breathing slowly in, breathing slowly out … And that as I slowly breathe in, then out, I am gently, safely, deeply, moving into a trance.

Now, I feel that stream of relaxation flowing from my legs, my pelvis, and into my abdomen, now into my back. I feel that stream of relaxation, flowing smoothly, gently, into my back. I am aware that with each breath in, and with each breath out, each vertebra becomes more and more relaxed … With each breath in, and with each breath out, each vertebra becomes more and more relaxed. Slowly out. I am feeling more and more relaxed. And as I feel more relaxed, and as my vertebrae feel gradually, one by one, relaxed, so I am aware that I am moving safely, gently, into a trance. As the relaxation flows into my back, into my vertebrae, I am aware how I am breathing slowly in, breathing slowly out … And that as I slowly breathe in, then out, I am gently, safely, deeply, moving into a trance.

Now I am aware that the stream of relaxation flowing through my body moves up into my shoulders and my neck. As I breathe slowly in, slowly out. Breathing in, breathing out, I feel my neck muscles, my shoulder muscles, becoming deeply relaxed … As I feel my neck, my shoulders feel slowly relaxed, I am aware that I am moving gently, deeply, safely into a trance ... Now I am aware that the relaxation is moving slowly up my neck, into my head, my face, my forehead, relaxing, deeply, and I am aware that as my head, my face, my forehead, get more relaxed, so I get deeper, deeper, into a trance. Across my forehead, into my face and the rest of my head, I feel this stream of relaxation. As I breathe in, and out, slowly, I feel my forehead, my face, my head, become deeply relaxed. Now I am aware of my eyelids feeling relaxed, deeply relaxed. They become gently, pleasantly heavy with relaxation. I am aware that as my eyelids relax, they become heavier, and heavier, pleasantly heavy, I can no longer keep them open ... As my eyelids close calmly and peacefully, I feel more and more relaxed, and as my eyes gently close, I am aware that I am moving deeper, and gently, into a trance ...

Nothing worries me. My eyes are closed; I feel relaxed. Now, the stream of relaxation is spreading slowly down my shoulders into the top of my right arm. Into my upper arm, past my elbow, into my forearm. My upper arm, my elbow, my forearm, slowly, deeply, becoming relaxed. First my upper arm. Then my elbow; the relaxation is spreading through down to my forearm. Then slowly, into my wrist, down into my hand, through my fingers. I am aware that my wrist, my hand, my fingers, right to the tips, are feeling deeply relaxed ...

Now, the stream of relaxation is spreading slowly down my shoulders into the top of my left arm. Into my upper arm, past my elbow, into my forearm. My upper arm, my elbow, my forearm, slowly, deeply, becoming relaxed. First my upper arm. Then my elbow; the relaxation is spreading through down to my forearm. Then slowly, into my wrist, into my hand, through my fingers. I am aware that my wrist, my hand, my fingers, right to the tips, are feeling deeply relaxed. As I breathe slowly, in, out ...

I am feeling deeply relaxed, and I am aware, now, that, as the relaxation grows, so I am moving deeper into a trance. My whole body feels relaxed, calm, at peace.

If by the end of this script there are parts of you that you feel need more relaxation then simply repeat the process as appropriate.

2. Reawakening
The way to reawaken or bring yourself out of a trance is as follows:
Now I begin to feel more awake and alert, bringing those positive feelings of relaxation with me as I become more aware of my surroundings. I will slowly count from one to five. With each number I will feel more and more alert. By the time I count five I will be wide awake, feeling alert and refreshed. One ... two ... three ... four ... five ...

3. Quitting Smoking
This script can be taped by you or someone else. At the end of the script, you can start the reawakening process. If you want to repeat it to yourself under hypnosis, rather than using a recording, simply change the text to first person, replacing "you are" with "I am."
You are now deep in a trance, deeply relaxed. I want you to think about your desires. About your desire to stop smoking. You want to ... stop smoking. You want to feel healthier ... you want to live longer, be fitter, be able to smell and taste, more ... You have smoked in the past when you have felt stressed, or under pressure ... You know you do not need to ... Smoking is something from your past, something you used to do, but you no longer have the desire to ... When in the future you feel stress or under pressure you will take five deep breaths ... slowly, and each time you breathe in, and breathe out, you will think of how healthy you feel, how good things smell ... That's good ...

You will notice how good it feels now, to have stopped smoking ... how much healthier you feel, because you know, really, you feel much better now, don't you, now that you are an ex-smoker? ... And you know, don't you, how good those five breaths feel each time, each time you feel under pressure, how healthy it feels? … You know that some of your friends smoke … but that is their problem, not yours, isn't it? … You do not mind their smoking, but you do not feel any urge to yourself … That's good, you feel better, don't you, knowing that you are in control of yourself now … how good it feels now that you have achieved your desire to stop smoking … how much better you are feeling already … and that as each day passes as an ex-smoker, you feel better … more healthy, more in control? You find it odd, don't you, that your friends smoke? But this does not worry you …you know you are an ex-smoker … That makes you feel good, doesn't it? I mean you are now in control, … and feeling healthier … better, healthier …

4. Overcoming Test Nerves

If you have studied hard but are worried that during the test your mind may go blank, you can use this script. At the end of the script, you can start the reawakening process.

Good. Now you are deeply relaxed. You feel good, you feel confident … I want you to imagine you are going to your test tomorrow; you feel confident … Imagine yourself sitting down at your desk, putting down your pens and pencils, that's right … see yourself with a quiet smile on your face, because you know, don't you, that you have studied hard? You know this stuff … Imagine too your test paper in front of you, and as you pick it up, confidently, to read it, a great sense of calmness settles upon you … You feel totally relaxed … Your mind is alert, ready for the questions … You know what to do … and as you start the test, as the signal is given, imagine yourself sitting there, able to recall all you need from those books, those notes … Good … You feel confident and calm, because you know, don't you, that you have studied hard? You know the answers; they come into your mind, naturally, don't they? … Your mind is calm and alert and focused on the test, isn't it? And you know that your unconscious, your mind, will be able to

remember the information you need, don't you, for your test, that you will be able to write it down? … And as you work through the test paper, you will be able, won't you, to answer each question you need to? You know it is all in your mind, that you can recall it … and that, when you have finished the test, you will feel quietly relaxed and calm … You know, don't you, that you will have done your best, that you will have answered all the questions you needed to, as well as you can? … You will continue to feel relaxed and calm… it's a good feeling, isn't it?

5. Helping Sleep

Try this script, or a variation of it, if you are having trouble getting to, or staying, asleep. At the end of the script, you can start the reawakening process.

That's good, it's nice, feeling relaxed, isn't it? … And when you are in bed, tonight, you may be aware of how relaxing it is, and then, because you are feeling relaxed, you may notice, that when you feel, deeply, relaxed, you feel sleepy … that your eyelids become heavier and heavier, your breath—can you hear it?—is getting deeper and deeper … and you may be aware that as you are feeling relaxed, in bed, you are feeling sleepier, and falling, asleep, gently … and then you sleep, deeply, peacefully, calmly, until your normal time to wake … awaking only if you need to, in deep sleep, and when you awake, normally, you may notice how you feel refreshed, relaxed … And you may be aware of feeling refreshed after you have slept deeply and peacefully … because in the end that's good, isn't it, going to bed, feeling relaxed, calm, and falling asleep, normally … knowing perhaps that each time you go to bed, to sleep, you may experience deep relaxation, and fall deeply asleep and stay peacefully asleep, awaking only if you need to, until your normal time to wake? … And, when you do awake, you may well think how refreshed and calm you feel, because you have slept so well … And it's good, feeling relaxed, falling asleep, waking refreshed …

Glossary

affect bridge The connection between your feeling/emotion now and the past incident that first provoked that feeling/emotion.

age progression Advancing a subject's age awareness during hypnosis so that he or she sees himself or herself in the future.

amnesia Loss of memory, which can occur when the subject is in a deep trance.

analgesia Removal of pain, but not of sensation.

anesthesia The absence of pain and sensation.

animal magnetism Mesmer's theory of a universal magnetic fluid that, when imbalanced within a person, causes illness that can be cured by a magnetic healer.

autohypnosis Self-hypnosis.

autonomic nervous system System controlling the unconscious functions of the body such as digestion, breathing, and heartbeat.

catalepsy Incapacitation of parts or all of the body during hypnotic trance.

confabulation The invention of "facts" to fill in gaps in memory.

deepening Helping the subject deeper into a trance with the use of words.

dissociation The splitting off from consciousness of certain ideas/emotions that then operate independently.

embedded suggestions The words/phrases that are placed in hypnotic inductions/scripts, and which emphasize the suggestion to the unconscious mind.

false-memory syndrome Where suggestions made or thoughts occurring to a subject during hypnosis appear, wrongly, to be real memories of actual events.

forensic hypnosis The use of hypnosis to help in investigations, for example in the interviewing of witnesses of crimes.

heterohypnosis Where hypnosis is induced in an individual by another.

hidden observer The idea that a part of our consciousness remains always aware of reality, even during a deep trance.

hypermnesia A vivid or complete memory of the past that occurs to the subject during hypnosis.

hypnotherapy The process of psychotherapy in which hypnosis is employed as part of the treatment.

ideomotor responses Where the muscles of a person in a trance respond involuntarily to an idea or feeling.

induction The process of helping a person into a hypnotic trance.

lay hypnotist Someone practicing hypnosis outside the medical profession.

monoideism The concept used by hypnosis pioneer James Braid to describe waking hypnosis and light stages of hypnosis.

neutral hypnosis The state where a person has been induced into a trance, but no suggestions have yet been made to the unconscious mind.

nocebo The opposite of a placebo, a nocebo is something that has no physical effect but which the subject believes will do him or her harm.

past-life regression Where patients are taken back in trance to supposed previous lives; most hypnotists regard these "memories" as useful metaphors occurring in the unconscious mind.

phobia Morbid, irrational fear of something.

placebo A substance of no medical effect given to patients who are told or believe it will do them good.

post-hypnotic suggestion A suggestion made during trance that influences or changes the subject's future behavior.

rapport When a hypnotist is in harmony or in tune with the subject and his or her unconscious mind.

reframing Seeing the world in a different way.

script The suggestions made to a person in a trance aimed at improving his or her life.

trance The state of altered consciousness that occurs during hypnosis, in which the hypnotist is able to communicate directly with the patient's unconscious mind.

trance logic During a trance the unconscious mind is able to accept suggestions/ideas even though they are (rationally) impossible and illogical.

Index

Page numbers in **bold** refer to boxes and timeline. Page numbers in *italics* refer to captions.

Resources

Internet
American Society of Clinical Hypnosis
http://www.asch.net

British Society of Clinical Hypnosis
http://www.bsch.org.uk

British Society of Medical and Dental Hypnosis
http://www.bsmdh.org

False-Memory Syndrome Foundation
http://www.fmsfonline.org

Hypnotherapy Society
http://www.hypnotherapysociety.com

James Braid Society
http://www.jamesbraidsociety.com/indexnew.htm

International Society of Hypnosis
http://www.ish.unimelb.edu.au/ish.html

Milton H. Erickson Foundation
http://www.erickson-foundation.org

Mindsci Clinic
http://www.mindsci-clinic.com

Society for Clinical and Experimental Hypnosis
http://ijceh.educ.wsu.edu

Books
Bandler, Richard *et al., Patterns of the Hypnotic Techniques of Milton H. Erickson, M.D.,* Metamorphous Press: US, 1997

Elman, Dave, *Hypnotherapy,* Westwood Publishing Company: US, 1984

Heller, Steven & Steele, Terry, *Monsters & Magical Sticks: There's No Such Thing As Hypnosis?,* New Falcon Publications: US, 2001

Hunter, Roy C., *Master the Power of Self-Hypnosis,* Sterling Publishing Company: US, 1998

James, Tad, *Hypnosis: A Comprehensive Guide,* Crown House Publishing: UK, 2000

Liggett, Donald R., *Sports Hypnosis,* Human Kinetics: US, 2000

Marshall-Warren, Deborah, *I'm Afraid of Hypnosis But I Don't Know Why,* Whole-Being Books: UK, 2003

McGill, Ormond, *The New Encyclopedia of Stage Hypnotism,* Crown House Publishing: US, 1996

Temes, Roberta, *The Complete Idiot's Guide to Hypnosis,* Alpha Books: US, 2000

Waterfield, Robin, *Hidden Depths: A History of Hypnosis,* Macmillan Publishing: UK, 2002

Credits
Special thanks to Dr. Chris Forester of the Hypnotherapy Society. Thanks also to Susan Rodgers of the American Society of Clinical Hypnosis, Barry Thain of Mindsci Clinic, and Tom Connelly of the British Society of Clinical Hypnosis.

Picture credits
Quarto would like to thank and acknowledge the following for supplying pictures reproduced in this book:
Key: l left, r right, c center, t top, b bottom

p6, p11t, p13tl, p14t, p15t, p16t, p18, p20t, p24t, p25tl, p26c, p28, p30t, p34, p73bl, p113, ANN RONAN LIBRARY / www.heritage-images.com / ISI
p7, Hulton-Deutsch Collection / CORBIS / ISI
p11b, p35, Topham Picturepoint / ISI
p22b, Cecil Beaton / CORBIS / ISI
p29, Courtesy of the Milton H. Erikson Foundation, Inc / ISI
p45b, p55, Bettmann / CORBIS
p59, Frank Trapper / CORBIS / ISI
p101t, Sergio Dorantes / CORBIS
p104, IMAGE STATE
p108t, H. Armstrong / CORBIS
p109, Hulton-Deutsch Collection / CORBIS
p110, Fin Costello / REDFERNS
p111, Roy Morsch / CORBIS
p112, Courtesy of Martin St. James and Quantum Entertainment / ISI
p115, Wand Enterprises / ISI
p121, Bettmann / CORBIS / ISI

All other photographs and illustrations are the copyright of Quarto Publishing plc. While every effort has been made to credit contributors, Quarto would like to apologize should there have been any omissions or errors.